Transforming Healthcare with Big Data and AI

A Volume in:
New Methods in the Era of Big Data and AI

Series Editor

Alex Liu
IBM

New Methods in the Era of Big Data and AI

Series Editor

Alex Liu
IBM

Transforming Healthcare with Big Data and AI

Edited by

Alex Liu
Atefeh (Anna) Farzindar
Mingbo Gong

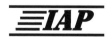

INFORMATION AGE PUBLISHING, INC.
Charlotte, NC • www.infoagepub.com

Library of Congress Cataloging-In-Publication Data

The CIP data for this book can be found on the Library of Congress website (loc.gov).

Paperback: 978-1-64113-897-0
Hardcover: 978-1-64113-898-7
E-Book: 978-1-64113-899-4

Printed in the United States of America

CONTENTS

TRANSFORMING HEALTHCARE WITH BIG DATA AND AI

Mingbo Gong

No one can talk about the development of human civilization without diving deep into the advancement of healthcare and medicine. Looking back at how today's healthcare system is shaped, there are many indispensable milestones. The practice of medicine began when Hippocrates of Kos started the first school of medicine, which established the medical profession and created the first document on the ethics of this profession. Galen of Pergamon was the first to apply anatomy to medicine, which influenced the development of anatomy and various healthcare fields.

The ten centuries between the fifth and the fifteenth century saw limited development in medicine and healthcare, and this period was filled with infectious and epidemic diseases. The development of healthcare and medicine finally saw the light, as Andreas Vesalius founded modern human anatomy in the sixteenth century. The next two centuries witnessed the discovery of microorganisms and the invention of the world's first vaccine in the eighteenth century.

With industrialization came an evolution of medicine and healthcare in the nineteenth century. Medical devices and technologies, such as x-rays, stethoscopes, sphygmomanometers, and thermometers were invented. Charles Darwin introduced the theory of evolution; Theodor Schwann extended cell theories; Florence Nightingale established the practice of nursing. Healthcare development

Transforming Healthcare with Big Data and AI, pages vii–viii.
Copyright © 2020 by Information Age Publishing
vii

did not slow down in the twentieth century with the world's first antibiotic substance, medical imageology, and molecular biology.

In the twenty-first century, more countries are considering healthcare as their top priority, computing and data storage capacities are increasing substantially, and more multi-disciplinary talents are coming into the healthcare industry. It is evident that the momentum of healthcare evolution will continue through the twenty-first century. We believe that the first two decades of the century will mark a new milestone in the history of healthcare, driven by the rapid development of health data and advanced data applications in healthcare.

How can we leverage data science and advanced data tools to advance the quality of our healthcare systems? This book aims to explore the critical topics at the intersection of data technologies and healthcare, with use cases and real-world examples that demonstrate how data science, artificial intelligence, IoT technologies, and blockchain are transforming healthcare.

This book is the fruit of a digital healthcare conference called Transforming Healthcare with Data, which took place on November 3, 2017, at the University of Southern California. Hosted by Mingbo Gong, Dr. Anna Farzinar, and Dr. Alex Liu, the conference invited 30 speakers and brought together over 300 healthcare practitioners, data technologists, civic leaders, researchers, and students. The conference was organized into three sessions: health data technologies, healthcare research, and digital health startups.

The health data technologies session covered popular topics in digital healthcare. The healthcare research session discussed how data science and open data are leveraged to advance healthcare research. The startup session invited founders of seven outstanding digital healthcare startups to demonstrate how their products are changing healthcare. One of the seven startups, Semioe Technology focuses on building semantic capacities into healthcare IoT in the Chinese market; another startup, Stasis Labs provides real-time monitoring systems in health facilities in India.

We are honored that many speakers of the conference decided to participate in the creation of this book. The authors make this book unique, as they come from multidisciplinary expertise as data scientists, healthcare experts, university professors, and entrepreneurs. This book can be used for educational and informational purposes by educators, healthcare practitioners, and data scientists, and it requires a basic technical background of data science and a general understanding of the healthcare industry.

CHAPTER 1

AN OVERVIEW

The Past, Present and Future
of Digital Health

Weixiang Chen

He who has Health has Hope; and he who has Hope has Everything.
                                                    —*Thomas Carlyle*

The healthcare industry is often referred to as a non-cyclical industry which is defined as an industry whose demand remains constant despite economic conditions. Simply put, healthcare is a necessity rather than a luxury. This status combined with the aging world population posits a rapid increase in healthcare expenditures for many countries including the United States.

In 2016, U.S. health spending accounted for 17.9 percent of the nation's GDP at $3.3 trillion, or $10,348 per person. This expenditure is projected to increase at an average rate of 5.5 percent per year from 2017 to 2026, reaching $5.7 trillion (19.7 percent of GDP) in 2026. From 1990 to 2007 the average annual growth rate was as high as 7.3 percent and decreased only slightly to 4.2 percent during the recession [1].

Projected national health spending and enrollment growth in healthcare services over the next decade is predominantly driven by fundamental economic and demographic factors: changes in projected income growth, increases in prices for

Transforming Healthcare with Big Data and AI, pages 1–20.
Copyright © 2020 by Information Age Publishing
1

medical goods and services, and enrollment shifts from private health insurance to Medicare which covers the aging population [2].

As healthcare expenditures increase, they will clearly become a more substantial burden on the budgets of states and families. To combat this growing crisis, new and innovative techniques must be developed. Increasing the efficiency of currently existing healthcare systems with the aid of technology is one of the few foreseeable solutions.

Technology-driven increases in healthcare efficiency may be achieved through telecommunication tools that enable virtual conversations between patients and providers, optimization of hospital management, data-driven decision support systems to facilitate doctors' work, or algorithm-assisted diagnosis and preventive care. Since most of these innovations involve digital tools, they are collectively referred to as "digital health."

According to the United States Food and Drug Administration (FDA), digital health encompasses innovations in both the hardware and software spaces [3]. Though these domains are classically distinct, growth in technology has blurred the border between them. For example, internet-of-things (IoT) devices such as wearables facilitate the collection of vast amounts of data, which is used as input for analytics software that utilizes machine learning and artificial intelligence (AI), whose predictions are subsequently used to improve the IoT devices. Other technologies in the digital health space include mobile health (mHealth), health information technology (IT), telehealth and telemedicine, and personalized medicine. This CHAPTER provides an overview of the digital health industry landscape through the lens of Big Data.

HISTORICAL AND TRADITIONAL USE OF DATA IN HEALTHCARE

The United States has been integrating data with healthcare, called Health Information Management (HIM) since 1928. In recent years, HIM innovations continue to affect the industry, primarily due to the implementation of electronic health records (EHR).

The HIM industry can trace its roots back to the 1920s, when healthcare professionals determined that documenting patient conditions benefited both providers and patients by establishing the details, complications, and outcomes of patient care. The practice of documentation became widely adopted after the healthcare industry concluded that a complete and accurate medical history was critical to the safety and quality of the patient experience.

The American College of Surgeons (ACOS) standardized these clinical records by establishing the American Association of Record Librarians, a professional association that exists today under the name American Health Information Management Association (AHIMA). These early medical records were documented on paper, which explains the name "record librarians."

1. The Evolution of Electronic Health Records (EHR)

Paper medical records have been maintained from the 1920s onward, but the technological advancements of the 60s and 70s introduced an innovative, computer-based information system. To ignite this growth, several pioneering American universities partnered with respected healthcare facilities to explore the potential for computers to revolutionize medical records. During these early experiments, patient information was generated and electronically recorded at a specific facility—and it was accessible only at that healthcare location, which restricted the software's usefulness. Other challenges during the early years of EHR included computer performance limitations and exorbitant pricing.

In the 1970s, the federal government began to integrate EHR with its pre-existing healthcare initiatives. The first widely adopted system was the Department of Veteran Affairs' implementation of VistA, known initially as the Decentralized Hospital Computer Program (DHCP) [4]. Technical aspects of healthcare software development had matured by the 1980s. The advent of computerized registration enabled patients to check in efficiently, and the introduction of the master patient index (MPI), a database of basic patient information used across all the departments of a healthcare organization, promoted a cross-departmental workflow to enhance the patient and caregiver experiences. These early successes encouraged individual hospital departments like Radiology and Laboratory to adopt specialized software systems, and computer healthcare applications began appearing on the market. The main limitation of the systems at the time was the lack of communication with each other or the capability to be accessed by neighboring departments, since the medical records for each department reside in data silos.

A spate of medical errors and patient deaths caused by healthcare providers prompted the search for a more viable EHR system in 2000. Electronic health records became the key to empower "providers to make better decisions and provide better care" while "reducing the incidence of medical error by improving the accuracy and clarity of medical records" [1]. President George W. Bush called for computerized health records in his 2004 State of the Union Address. A modern EHR revolution had begun.

Present-day healthcare organizations are implementing functional EHR systems at a faster rate than ever, largely due to President Obama's passage of the American Recovery and Reinvestment Act (ARRA) in 2009. ARRA "requires the adoption of Electronic Medical Records by 2014 for seventy percent of the primary care provider population," according to the US Department of Health and Human Services. This requirement has led the Office of the National Coordinator for Health Information Technology to establish 62 Regional Extension Centers (RECs) across the nation [5]. These RECs offer support to healthcare providers as they adopt electronic health records and transition towards a universal EHR system.

2. HIPAA Regulations

The wide adoption of EHR enabled efficient sharing and transfer of medical records, but it also introduced privacy and security risks. Before the early 1990s, only a patchwork of federal and state laws governed the transfer of personal health information. Unfortunately, these laws were inconsistent in their regulation of health information transmission, resulting in loopholes that allowed personal health information to be transferred for non-medical purposes. To combat privacy breaches, the Health Insurance Portability and Accountability Act (HIPAA) was established and signed into law in 1996 to protect individual patient information.

HIPAA restricts the use of Big Data in digital health. Data-sharing is critical to effective utilization of Big Data in all domains, but HIPAA regulations, while essential for ensuring consumer privacy, heavily restrict the dynamism of data-sharing in healthcare. Thus, it is crucial for digital health professionals to familiarize themselves with HIPAA and its intricacies.

HIPAA is divided into five Titles. Title I of HIPAA protects health insurance coverage for workers and their families when they change or lose their jobs. Title II of HIPAA, known as the Administrative Simplification (AS) provisions, requires the establishment of national standards for electronic healthcare transactions and national identifiers for providers, health insurance plans, and employers. Title III sets guidelines for pre-tax medical spending accounts, Title IV sets guidelines for group health plans, and Title V governs company-owned life insurance policies [6]. Below is a summary of the main HIPAA regulations that are most relevant to digital health professionals.

The HIPAA Privacy Rule defines protected health information (PHI) as individually identifiable health information that is held or maintained by a covered entity such as health plans, healthcare clearinghouses, and healthcare providers. PHI includes demographic information, information about the patient's physical or mental condition, genetic information, and information about the patient's healthcare plan or payment system. The Privacy Rule mandates that appropriate safeguards be implemented to protect the privacy of PHI. When patient authorization is not obtained, the Privacy Rule sets limits and conditions regarding the use and disclosure of PHI.

The HIPAA Security Rule contains the national standards that must be met to protect electronic PHI (ePHI). The Security Rule applies to any system or individual who has access to confidential patient data. Access is defined as having the means to read, write, modify, or communicate ePHI or personal identifiers that may reveal the identity of the patient. There are three subsections within the Security Rule: Technical Safeguards, Physical Safeguards, and Administrative Safeguards. Each aspect comes with a series of regulations, some of which are required for all covered entities, while others are considered "addressable" that allow more flexibility with respect to compliance. Finally, the HIPAA Breach Notification Rule requires covered entities to inform patients when their PHI has been compromised. If the breach affects more than 500 patients, covered entities must promptly notify the HHS (The U.S. Department of Health and Human Services) and issue a notice to the media.

In summary, the HIPAA rules are a set of regulations concerning the collection, usage, storage and transfer of electronic healthcare records. These rules are especially applicable when the data are personally identifiable information, which may cause certain health information to be linked to individual patients. Therefore, unlike many other digital sectors which readily collect, analyze, and even sell personal information (such as the social media and e-commerce domains), any privacy-related healthcare data is to be strictly regulated under HIPAA. This restricts the rapid and widespread adoption of data usage in the healthcare industry and creates a barrier of entry to non-healthcare participants.

DIGITAL HEALTH: A FLOURISHING NEW SECTOR

The answer is the disruptive innovator, an outsider, who creates a product or services...

—*Clayton Christensen, The Innovator's Dilemma (1997)*

The healthcare industry's distinct combination of ubiquity and conservatism encourage its disruption by outsider innovations. The creation of "digital health" via the coupling of computerized healthcare tools such as EHR with Big Data and AI has vastly increased opportunities for technologists to make an impact on healthcare.

1. Technology Corporations and Healthcare

The advent of a new era in digital health is heralded by technology corporations such as Google and Apple, who are currently increasing research and development expenditures in digital health. These companies have not been traditionally active in healthcare.

Google made headlines in January 2014 when it announced that, for the past eighteen months, it had been working on a contact lens that could help diabetic people by continually checking their glucose levels. At the end of 2015, Google partnered with the digital health company Dexcom to launch a new generation of continuous glucose monitors.

But Google's ambition in healthcare goes beyond medical devices. Google's Calico project, for example, is a high-tech research and development lab that aims to combat aging. Google's life sciences department, Verily is yet another example. Led by famous cell biologist Andy Conrad, Verily has some futuristic projects lined up that could change healthcare forever. For example, "Project Baseline" is a broad effort designed to develop a clear reference, or baseline, of good health and a data-rich platform that can be used to better identify risk factors for diseases. Partnering with Duke University and Stanford Medicine to collect, organize and analyze broad phenotypic health data from approximately ten thousand participants, Google is leveraging its capability to manage and understand large datasets to shift the healthcare sector from a "disease-centric" philosophy to a "health-centric" philosophy.

Another technology giant, Apple is not far behind Google in offering a range of new products and services. The Apple Watch, for example, tracks the user's daily habits, heartbeat, activity levels and more. Apple's HealthKit is an Internet platform that can store data from different devices, such as the Apple Watch, and share it with a user's healthcare provider. In addition, Apple's ResearchKit (launched in 2015) and the CareKit (launched in 2016) are open-source frameworks that allow developers to build healthcare apps. In the past decade, Apple has established itself as one of the dominant players pushing innovation in healthcare.

IBM has also made headlines in healthcare news. In April 2015, IBM revealed its commitment to improving healthcare with the launch of the supercomputer IBM Watson Health and the Watson Health Cloud platform. By leveraging Watson's powerful machine learning and cloud computing capabilities, IBM has the opportunity to make a significant impact on digital health. By 2018, IBM Watson Health had engineered several key deals, including the acquisition of Merge Healthcare and various other strategic partnerships. Notable among these are IBM Watson Health's partnerships with Apple, to analyze its ResearchKit data; with CVS Health, to transform care management for patients with chronic diseases; and with Johnson & Johnson, to develop new drugs. IBM Watson Health also collaborates with the American Diabetes Association (ADA) to develop a diabetes advising system for patients and caregivers. Finally, among many other initiatives in cancer, diabetes, and other diseases, IBM has also announced the formation of a new Watson Health medical imaging collaborative platform.

What caused this sudden influx of corporate interest in digital health? Healthcare had not always been a favorite topic for IT companies, but the rapid changes in the industry have made business justifications easier. Healthcare has always been a sensitive and largely complex universe. The industry is begging for innovative solutions that can make healthcare easier to navigate—for both patients and providers. The fact that healthcare in the United States alone is worth $3 trillion makes it obviously attractive to tech companies who want a piece of the profits.

But future collaborations between technology corporations and healthcare professionals are not going to be without rocky patches. The healthcare field is conservative for a reason—it is one of the most tightly regulated industries because of its relationship to human health, individual privacy, and data concerns. If a consumer website is down for an hour, it is probably not the end of the world; if a life-maintaining medical device malfunctions for just minutes, a patient's life can be at risk. Besides, health services and specialty devices are not readily allowed to be sold directly to consumers without FDA approval like ordinary consumer goods, and the interplay among the regulators, providers (doctors and hospitals), payors (health insurance) and patients is often more complicated than a simple consumer relationship. Overestimating consumers' willingness to use technology to monitor their daily activities, failure to fully understand patient-clinician relationships, and ignoring regulatory procedures are some of the other hurdles that the tech giants face in healthcare projects.

The advent of digital health under major technology corporations may be just what the field needs to kick start a period of explosive growth.

2. Creating the Ecosystem: Building Community and Modern Healthcare Communications

Technology corporations in healthcare not only bring an outsider's view to the digital health field, but also a vast amount of capital. For example, Google Ventures, the investment arm of the search engine giant, deploys more than one-third of its investments in the life science sector and is ranked a leading investor in the digital health field. The total for digital health funding in 2014 more than doubled compared to 2013 and is almost six times the amount invested in 2010. Figure 1.1 shows the trend of this massive influx of money up to the first half of 2018 [7].

Venture capital money nourishes a very diversified digital health ecosystem. In these early phases, many startups are coming into the healthcare industry by making "peripheral changes," or trying to bring the healthcare sector up to date on a par with other fields. Typical innovations at this stage include healthcare-focusing social media websites, online communities, telecommunication tools that enable faster connection between doctors and patients, and online doctors' appointment

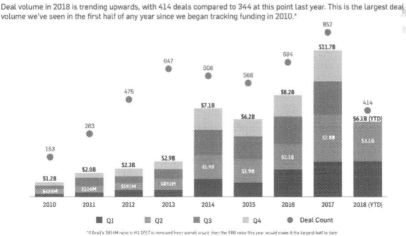

FIGURE 1.1. Deal Volumes in Digital Healthcare

sites. Similar tools or websites have been well established for almost ten years for other uses (for example, LinkedIn was founded in 2002 and Facebook in 2004); therefore, these notable healthcare-focusing startups are just a reflection of the conservative nature of the industry.

Below, we take a look at some of the typical digital health startups that made news between 2014–2017 (the funding summary of the companies are based on open information from Crunchbase).

Doximity, the "LinkedIn for doctors," is an online social network platform for healthcare professionals founded in 2011. As of late 2018, it claims to have covered over 70% of US doctors and 45% of all nurse practitioners and physician assistants as verified members. The company was inspired by the massive increase in demand for doctors and health care services under the Affordable Care Act, when millions of uninsured Americans entered the healthcare system for the first time. While building the online community for medical professionals to enable faster connection between peers, the company also offers specialized tools needed by doctors, such as continuing education credits, ability to send/fax HIPAA-compliant messages or medical figures, medical job postings, and research literature alerts. Doximity successfully raised a total of $81.8M in funding and reached a positive cash flow in January 2014, before its April 2014 Series C funding round led by DFJ and Morgan Stanley.

MyHealthTeams is a social network site for people with chronic conditions such as autism, breast cancer, COPD, Lupus, and multiple sclerosis. Founded in 2012, it has reached up to 1.5 million people across thirteen countries and currently covers twenty-nine conditions. The company believes that when people facing the same chronic condition can connect with and learn from each other, ask questions, get referrals and share tips with others, health outcomes improve.

PatientsLikeMe started with a similar idea of building an online network of people with similar chronic disease but went one step further. Founded in 2004, PatientsLikeMe not only allows patients to connect with each other, but it also encourages them to share symptoms, treatment information, and health outcomes. This allows the company to aggregate millions of data points about diseases so that they can analyze and reveal new insights. These data and patient experiences are also shared with the healthcare industry to develop better products, services, and care. The company claims to have helped epilepsy patients improve their self-management and self-efficacy, helped the FDA gain new insights into drug safety, and even refuted clinical trial results based on the peer-to-peer network's real-time evaluation of treatment. The company has become the world's largest personalized health network.

PillPack is an "online pharmacy" company founded in 2013. The company offers a full-service, licensed online pharmacy that aims to make the management of prescriptions and medications easier for customers. Medication is sorted by the dose into individual packets to help patients stay on track, delivery is sent directly to the door, and the platform works with doctors to automatically manage refills. Essentially, PillPack is aiming to be the Amazon of medical prescriptions. The company has raised about $118M in funding through their Series D round in 2016.

Kareo belongs to another category of startups aiming to help doctors simplify their small practice by offering cloud-based practice management software. Tools include HIPAA-compliant administrative software replacing paperwork, billing services, telecommunication or other patient engagement tools, revenue analytic, and others. In all, the company helps individual practice doctors keep track of the fast changes in healthcare and embrace a more digitalized practice, allowing them more time to work with patients.

ZocDoc is another successful digital health startup aiming to provide online booking of doctors' appointments. Patients can see real-time availability of doctors, confirm who accepts their insurance plan and read feedback and reviews of doctors from other patients. On the healthcare side, the platform integrates with doctors' calendars in real-time and helps tap into the hidden supply of medical providers' availabilities, such as the ten to twenty percent of medical appointments that are canceled or rescheduled at the last minute. Other functions include doctor's profiles and ratings, waiting room forms submission, and more. It has attracted renowned investors such as the Founders Fund, DST, Goldman Sachs, and Amazon CEO Jeff Bezos.

In summary, during this early development phase, many of the digital health startups are streamlining various aspects of the healthcare industry with modern digital tools. They may seem to be just an extension of the well-established group of internet companies, but they are addressing some of the most important challenges in healthcare. Today's product manufacturers or service providers can easily connect to their consumers via the internet, but it is an entirely different story when it comes to doctors and patients. The healthcare industry cannot avoid catering to doctors' needs. Doctor's expertise also cannot be easily replaced.

Digitalization tools are tapping into the convenience aspect before additional technological advancements make major disruptions in other areas of the healthcare industry.

3. Data-Driven Innovations: Clinical Trials, R&D, and Wearables

Digital tools improve communications in healthcare. However, they do not necessarily change much of the essence of the field—health and disease are still diagnosed manually by human doctors, based on conventional information and methods. The "peripheral changes" are exciting for the healthcare industry, but the excitement was quickly eclipsed by the fundamental changes driven by newer technologies like big data and artificial intelligence.

The term "Big Data" has been in use since the 1990s [8]. A milestone of the industry was the release of MapReduce, the parallel processing model developed by Google in 2004. Machine-learning driven artificial intelligence showed its power in solving complicated problems using massive amounts of data. Big data and

AI have been a hot topic that drives innovations in various fields since the beginning of the century, before they finally found their way into healthcare and digital health in less than a decade. Let's look at some of the applications below.

(1) Clinical Trials

A clinical trial is such an essential part of the development of a new drug or device that it can account for forty percent of a typical pharma research budget. The process is slow, expensive, and includes a lot of bookkeeping. Every year in the U.S., approximately two million patients participate in roughly 3000 clinical trials; up to ninety percent of trials are delayed or over budget. There is room for improvement in almost every step of these clinical trials by using big data and AI technologies.

Finding and recruiting the right patient for a matching clinical trial is the first step. For example, a principal investigator for a non-small cell lung cancer trial using traditional recruitment methods can spend six months to validate twenty-three eligible patients for a biomarker. In comparison, Deep 6 AI, a startup established in 2015, found and validated fifty-eight eligible matches in less than ten minutes by using AI to mine medical records and to accelerate finding and recruiting patients for clinical trials. Less than five percent of cancer patients enroll in a clinical trial, often because patients and doctors don't know what trials are available, compared to the 25%–50% of cancer patients which should have been enrolled to hasten cures for cancer. Deep 6 AI uses Natural Language Processing (NLP) to read doctors' notes, pathology reports, diagnosis, recommendations, and to detect lifestyle data, such as smoking and activity history. It then graphs this information and matches appropriate patients with clinical trial criteria, potentially reducing recruitment time from years to just days or weeks. The company also uses fuzzy matching to detect patients with undiagnosed symptoms and characteristics, such as cognitive decline or chronic pain. This allows sponsors who want to test new drugs for Alzheimer's, chronic pain, or other disorders to find symptomatic and undiagnosed patients, and in turn, it offers patients the opportunities to be informed about new trial studies.

During an ongoing clinical trial, AI can predict which patients have a higher chance of dropping out or not following protocols using algorithms based on both historical and incoming data throughout the trial. Then clinicians can track patients individually, and send reminders to take medications at specific times, submit forms, or keep appointments. Technologies such as digital reporting apps, as well as wearables, also allow for real-time engagement and communication to support patient-centric trials. Patients can send feedback on treatment reactions, manage medication intake, and share information with researchers, reducing or eliminating the need for patients to travel to sites, which increases patient adherence and compliance. It is noteworthy to point out that AI-driven customer engagement is a well-established method used in internet companies. Startups such as Trials.AI are tailoring this technique to clinical trials and have reported ninety-eight percent patient adherence.

AI technologies also offer better measurements of treatment outcomes. For example, in the treatment of Alzheimer's disease, trial researchers rely heavily on verbal or written evidence from patient visits and direct clinic observations to assess patient progress, but subjective evidence can be unreliable and may not provide enough information for decision making. Startups like WinterLight Labs use quantifiable data from algorithms to decipher subtle patterns beyond human perception by measuring thousands of variations in voice patterns, including pitch, frequency, amplitude, grammar idiosyncrasies, subject matter, and its emotional impact on the patient.

It is unwise to ignore the potential contribution in this field by existing technology corporations. As mentioned above, Google's Project Baseline is one example aiming to collect and analyze data for over 10,000 healthy individuals to map out a baseline for "healthy." Apple's ResearchKit directly serves healthcare researchers, while HealthKit and CareKit will also be gathering valuable information about human health. These will also contribute to a better understanding of health and disease.

(2) Medical R&D and Drug Development

In addition to clinical research, big data and AI will have a lot to contribute to the fields of drug development and medical R&D. Drug development is inefficient and expensive, due to high development costs (around $2 billion for a newly approved treatment) and low clinical trial success rates (below twelve percent). About fifteen to twenty percent of the development costs are in the discovery phase, which can take hundreds of millions of dollars. Reducing the cost and time of drug discovery is as imperative as increasing the clinical trial success rate.

Computer simulations have been used in drug development since the 1990s. From compound screening, molecule designing, potency and toxicity prediction to disease target identification, data technologies are adding to the power of the traditional simulation. Drug discovery often involves identifying hidden patterns in large volumes of data, where AI technologies such as machine learning excel.

For example, a biotech company founded in 2006 called Berg is focusing on therapeutic discovery using its unique AI-based platform. This platform combines patient biology and artificial intelligence-based analytics to explore the differences between healthy and diseased environments, with the goal of discovery and development of drugs, diagnostics and healthcare applications. The company has developed a model to identify previously unknown cancer mechanisms using tests on more than 1,000 cancerous and healthy human cell samples. They modeled diseased human cells by varying the levels of sugar and oxygen the cells were exposed to, and then tracked their lipid, metabolite, enzyme and protein profiles. The group uses its AI platform to generate and analyze immense amount of biological and outcomes data from patients to highlight critical differences between diseased and healthy cells [9]. Ultimately, the employment of AI translates to faster discovery and development of treatments, a reduction in costs, and more effective precision treatments for individuals.

Big data and AI technologies are also helping researchers understand background information before they start on a drug development process. A London-based startup called BenevolentBio has its own AI platform which is fed data from sources such as research papers, patents, clinical trials, and patient records. This forms a representation based in the cloud, of more than one billion known and inferred relationships between biological entities such as genes, symptoms, diseases, proteins, tissues, species and candidate drugs. This data is then processed to produce a 'knowledge graph' (which works almost like a search engine that depicts the relationship between core concepts) of, for example, a medical condition and its associated genes, or the compounds that have been shown to affect it. The platform uses natural language processing to recognize entities and understand their links to other things. "AI can put all this data in context and surface the most salient information for drug-discovery scientists," says Jackie Hunter, chief executive of BenevolentBio [9]. The company was founded in 2013 and has secured $207M in funding up to 2018.

Machine learning and other AI technologies have been used in various aspects of the drug development process to: aggregate and synthesize information, understand mechanisms of disease, generate data and models, repurpose existing drugs, generate novel drug candidates, validate drug candidates, design drugs, design and run preclinical experiments, design recruit and optimize clinical trials, publish data, etc. There are hundreds of companies that are working in this field, from big pharma investing heavily into AI-driven drug discoveries to startups in all phases [10].

(3) Wearables and Internet of Things (IoT) Devices

The health IoT startup is an interesting and unique category as they leverage both hardware and software. Wearable devices enable collection of additional information about health from both patients and healthy individuals. The real-time information about human bodies will almost certainly lead to new insights into health and disease. Investor interest in healthcare IoT startups has grown together with the broader boom in digital health that increased twenty percent in 2015 [11].

The boom in wearables started with hardware startups that provide activity monitoring, such as Fitbit, Jawbone, and more. These consumer products can track daily activities and sleep patterns with wristbands, headsets, and other articles. Increasingly, IoT startups are developing new healthcare applications and are leveraging connected sensors to better diagnose, monitor, and manage patients and treatment. Many companies are focusing on clinical-grade wearables to track patient data more robustly, while others see opportunities to establish sensor networks within health facilities to optimize healthcare monitoring and delivery.

Interestingly, the application of wearable IoT devices is driving changes in the payor (insurance) sector as well. Conventionally, health insurance companies calculate the risk of a customer based on population statistics such as gender, age, medical history, and other factors. Empowered by the personalized information collected by the wearables, the payor now has a much better chance to understand the customer's daily habits. Large insurance companies like United Health are already offering programs encouraging participants to use wearable devices for step tracking. When they reach daily walking targets, financial incentives up to $1460 per year are provided. In this way, participants keep themselves healthier saving the payor much more in medical costs [12].

Based on the purposes of the wearables, health IoT companies can be roughly broken down into the following categories [11]:

- **Clinical efficiency:** using connected objects to improve the delivery of healthcare in hospitals and clinics, and track treatments to boost the effectiveness of healthcare providers. Some companies use smart glass wearables like Google Glass for healthcare charting. Some harness the Apple Watch so doctors can track patient visits and access EMRs. Others use IoT sensors for location-tracking on patients and medical equipment in real-time, such as an internet-connected pill bottle that monitors medicine adherence.
- **Clinical-grade biometric sensors and wearables:** companies focus on connected biometric sensors for use in a clinical or hospital setting, and some companies in patient care (such as EarlySense and Monica Healthcare) have FDA approval. Others offer clinical IoT equipment for diagnosis such as vision testing.
- **Consumer and home monitoring:** companies develop technology marketed to consumers for the collection of biometric information, such as addiction cessation trackers, smart thermometers, biometric trackers for glucose levels, and more. This category also includes monitoring systems like Qardio and AliveCor, which allow for ECG (electrocardiogram) testing to be done from home.
- **Brain sensors and neurotechnology**: this category is mostly comprised of startups trying to "hack the brain" with high-tech consumer-targeted cranial wearables. For example, headbands that read brainwaves, and devices that transmit mood-elevating neuro signals. This space includes clinical-grade projects focused on noninvasive neurotech (brain wave reading/recording) to analyze drug efficacy and track neuropathology.
- **Fitness wearables and sleep monitoring:** including startups focusing on fitness tracking consumer wearables, smart apparel, and wristbands to detect sleep patterns and other daily habits.
- **Infant monitoring:** wearable technology that monitors infant movements and vitals.

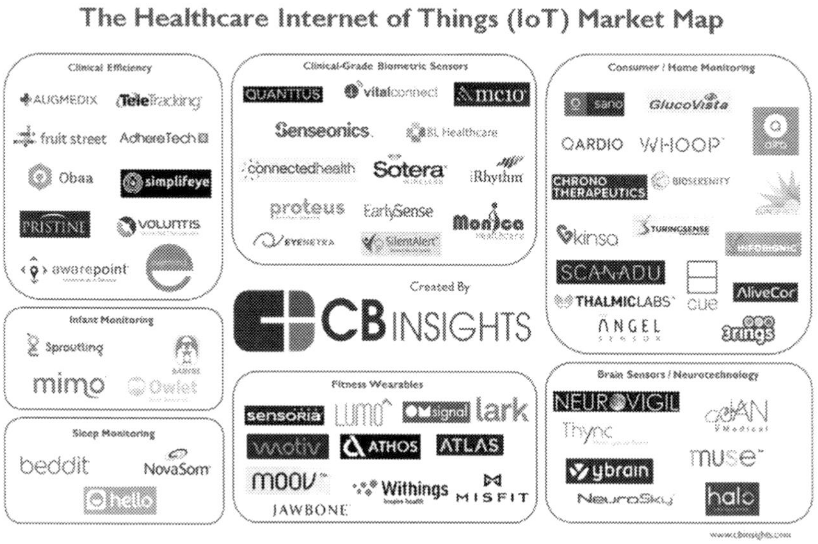

The Healthcare Internet of Things (IoT) Market Map

FIGURE 1.2. Wearable IoT Startups

Wearable IoT startups make up a good percentage of the companies in the digital health field. Figure 1.2 shows some example of the distinguished names in this sector (2016).

For many consumer-grade wearable companies, data quality and user adherence are among the biggest challenges to their success. Reports show that more than fifty percent of consumers lose interest and stop wearing the device after a few months [13]. Ensuring long-term engagement remains a crucial problem to be solved. However, with more clinical-grade IoT devices or applications being developed, and the value from these data proven and widely accepted, data-driven health IoTs are a trend that is not to be underestimated in the future of digital health.

Above, we summarized some of the ongoing efforts in the digital health sector. There are many more exciting things to be done to improve the field, which may disrupt the healthcare industry in a way that we cannot imagine today.

THE FUTURE GOAL FOR DIGITAL HEALTH: BETTER HEALTH AT AN AFFORDABLE PRICE

Two core values of the healthcare industry are: diagnosing and treating diseases and keeping people healthy in the first place. However, the diagnosis and treatment processes are almost entirely manual and wholly dependent on doctors' personal experience, which is so inconsistent that it becomes the bottleneck of the industry. If we can't significantly increase the efficiency of these steps, offering affordable healthcare to everybody, everywhere is far-fetched.

Diagnosis is essentially a deduction process based on very complicated information, considering that the secrets of health and disease are not fully understood yet. In the US, it typically takes seven to eleven years of medical school and residency to train an MD for medical licensing, then years if not decades of actual clinical experience for them to become domain experts. Expert doctors are always in short supply, making equal healthcare for everyone unrealistic.

Luckily, computers and artificial intelligence are especially good at information processing and deduction. In recent years, the most exciting progress in the digital health field is undoubtedly AI-driven diagnosis and wellness tools that tap right into the core of healthcare: how to diagnose and treat, and how to keep people healthy.

1. AI-Driven Diagnosis

(1) Image diagnostic tools

April 11, 2018 marked the beginning of a new era when the FDA approved the world's first AI diagnostic device, produced by a company called IDx [14]. The IDx-DR, a software program that uses an artificial intelligence algorithm to analyze images of the eye taken with a retinal camera. It's used to detect greater than a mild level of the eye disease diabetic retinopathy, which causes vision loss and affects thirty million people in the US.

In practice, a doctor uploads the digital images of the patient's retinas to a cloud server on which IDx-DR software is installed. The software provides the doctor with one of two results: (1) "more than mild diabetic retinopathy detected: refer to an eye care professional" or (2) "negative for more than mild diabetic retinopathy; rescreen in 12 months." If a positive result is detected, patients should see an eye care provider for further diagnostic evaluation and possible treatment as soon as possible.

IDx-DR is the first authorized device that provides a screening decision without the need for a clinician to interpret the image or results, making it usable by healthcare providers who are typically not involved in eye care. Although results tell only whether a patient needs additional diagnoses from an eye care professional, it still marks the dawn of a new era where AI algorithms are (partially) replacing human doctors for professional opinions.

IDx-DR software is taking advantage of the image processing algorithms of artificial intelligence. Significant progress has been made in this area during the recent decade because of increased data availability, more powerful processing, and more sophisticated algorithms like deep learning. Deep learning is a category of machine learning based on artificial neural networks, which has been an area of academic research since the 1940s. Due to recent advancement in GPU processing power and the faster accumulation of (labeled) images from the internet, deep learning has become the top technique for effective machine learning. Deep learning started to exert its real power with corporations like Google announcing the wide applications of deep learning in face recognition, image processing, and voice recognition. In March 2016, Google's AlphaGo program, a Go-playing AI based on deep learning, beat the world champion Lee Sedol in a five-game match. Only two decades ago, when IBM's chess program Deep Blue beat the world champion Garry Kasparov, the New York Times proclaimed that "it may be a hundred years before a computer beats humans at Go — maybe even longer," because the Go game has more possible moves than the number of atoms in the observable universe. The astonishingly rapid development of deep learning techniques brings significant advancement in image recognition applications, enabling not only enables companies like Google and Facebook to build applications that distinguish Chihuahuas from muffins, but also finding value in medical diagnosis.

Healthcare image diagnostic tools have been developed in many verticals in healthcare, with a steady increase in diagnostic accuracy and sensitivity. Cancer cells, for example, can be detected by a trained system that analyzes images of human tissues. Google has announced the capability to detect breast cancer at an AUC (area under the curve, which is the average value of sensitivity for all possible values of specificity) of as high as 0.98 and to detect prostate cancer at an AUC of 0.96 [15]. In contrast, an average well-trained human pathologist has an average of seventy percent accuracy. In another report, dermatology researchers from Germany have developed an algorithm that successfully detects 95% of melanomas from skin cancer images, in contrast with 86.6% by human dermatologists [16].

Tech companies are rapidly implementing deep learning tools in real clinical settings, and the types of disease that can be diagnosed using image processing tools are also expanding. Imagine a future where a patient can go to a nearby imaging clinic (or maybe use a smartphone) to take medical images then upload it to the cloud for an instant diagnosis with accuracy higher than any human doctors at a fraction of the price. Healthcare will be truly affordable and equal for everybody then.

It is true that AI-driven image diagnostic tools are not without limitations at this stage. For example, questions have been raised regarding the absence of extensive clinical trials, the lack of peer reviews, and the potential errors resulting from improper learning samples [17]. But all modern technologies in their infancy need room to improve before being fully embraced. Given enough time, AI-based image diagnostic software will be one of the first tools to fundamentally disrupt the medical industry.

(2) IBM Watson

IBM has recently scaled up its commitment to digital health, and its effort mainly revolves around their AI called Watson. IBM's approach to digital health is unique, so it is worth a brief discussion.

Watson made its debut by winning the Jeopardy game against human champions in 2011 using its advanced natural language processing (NLP) and search tree capabilities [18]. IBM added to the core NLP capabilities other data processing tools such as visualization dashboards and statistical models. They are marketing Watson as an AI tool that can interact with users in human languages and answer questions about complicated problems automatically.

Watson is adapted to offer cancer treatment plans by taking in thousands of medical publications, clinical trials, and doctors' notes so that it can organize suggestions to human oncologists in human-readable languages. The idea is that the AI's processing power allowed it to consider all the available research papers or clinical trials that the human oncologists might not have read at the time of diagnosis.

In 2016, researchers at the University of North Carolina School of Medicine tested Watson by having the AI analyze 1,000 cancer diagnoses. In ninety-nine percent of the cases, Watson was able to recommend treatment plans that matched actual suggestions from oncologists. Furthermore, Watson found treatment options human doctors missed in thirty percent of the cases [19]. Watson has partnered with major cancer hospitals and medical facilities like Quest Diagnostics and MD Anderson Cancer Center, although the latter terminated their partnership in 2017 due to "too high costs with unsatisfying results." In 2018, various partners accused Watson of "giving unsafe recommendations" in treating cancer. Questions have been raised as to whether Watson, once praised as the future of cancer research, has fallen far short of expectations [20].

There are many reasons that Watson hasn't exactly lived up to its lofty expectations, such as the overclaim in the marketing messages, the mismatch between the "learning samples" and real patient data, the ongoing research and development, etc. After all, any claims that an in-development AI can be as good as humans in solving complicated problems like cancer which are not fully understood yet is probably an overreach. But undoubtedly IBM is continuing to improve its AI capabilities in health diagnosis.

Only time will tell what kinds of diagnostic applications technology will bring us to one day—something that we may not even imagine as of now. It is beyond doubt that such tools and AI capabilities will be of enormous benefit to patients around the world.

(3) AI-Driven Preventive Care

Besides AI-based diagnostic tools, AI-driven preventive care is another futuristic application that is showing early promise.

Western medical philosophy is based on a "disease-centric" approach, where research and medical services focus on diagnosing and treating the disease after it occurs. However, with the advancement in holistic medicine—a healing philosophy that considers the whole person (body, mind, spirit, and emotions) in the quest for optimal health and wellness, and with the increasing cost of healthcare, the shift in emphasis toward a "wellness" approach is becoming more accepted.

While the country's payor system is transitioning from a fee-for-service model to a value-based model, it calls for a healthcare system that is preventive rather than reactionary. This transition is especially valuable for chronic disease conditions, which account for approximately seventy-five percent of the nation's aggregate health spending [21]. Today, patients diagnosed with chronic conditions such as cancer or diabetes often realize it too late to reverse the progression of the disease. Treatment plans for late-stage illnesses can also be costly and often unproductive. If patients can be better equipped with insights into their health, they would be able to make healthier lifestyle choices and better adhere to physician advice and therefore have better outcomes. Consequently, preventing the start of chronic disease and managing the disease early on has become the focus of preemptive measures in healthcare.

Chronic conditions like COPD and congestive heart failure often show early signs, which AI can detect based on key biometric information. Companies like Sentrian (founded in 2012) are using IoT devices to track patient conditions in real-time and predict whether the disease will progress. Preventive interventions can be introduced early on and reduce preventable hospitalizations. The company has reported a 2–3 times improvement over the current remote patient monitoring systems.

AI-driven disease prediction is also being developed in other fields. For example, researchers from Sutter Health and the Georgia Institute of Technology are using deep learning to analyze electronic health records to predict heart failure before it happens. Initial results have demonstrated that this AI application can accurately predict heart failure one to two years early. Philadelphia's Thomas Jefferson University Hospital has researchers training AI to identify tuberculosis on chest X-rays, an initiative which may help screening and evaluation efforts in TB-prevalent areas where access to radiologists is limited [22].

AI healthcare startups that are working with predictive and preventive medicine are on the rise. Out of 218 healthcare AI startups selected from a startup database, fifty-four were involved in predictive medicine, with forty-four founded in 2010 or later [23]. Although it will take time for the healthcare industry to fully embrace AI-driven preventive care models, AI is already accelerating the speed at which we understand diseases and treat them more efficiently at a lower cost.

FINAL THOUGHTS

In this chapter, we outlined the history and current development of how data and digital tools are transforming healthcare. We began with the establishment of EHR systems and HIPAA regulations, and then we introduced the digital evolutions that aim to improve the efficiency of healthcare operations. We dived deep into how big data and artificial intelligence are driving fundamental changes in healthcare by disrupting healthcare processes, such as clinical trials, drug developments, diagnoses, and disease treatment. With the rapid growth of digital health in both academic research and industrial applications, this chapter is nowhere near a complete depiction of the vast amount of disruptive innovations of the sector; it only aims to provide an outline of the picture.

It is becoming clear that while data and AI technologies are making incremental changes in healthcare, they are ready to bring more disruptions into how humans and machines interact in the sector. Although doctors still play the most significant role in healthcare, machines that can perform operations and provide assessment will become more widely adopted. Are doctors one day going to be replaced by computers and machines? Not likely anytime soon, but with the pace that technology is evolving, we should always keep an open mind, especially since AI algorithms have surpassed human doctors in several areas of health diagnostics.

With the United States healthcare system transitioning into a value-based payer model, big data and AI is driving the health industry into a preventive care system. It is only a matter of time until this "health-centric" philosophy will become more prevalent than the traditional "disease-centric" philosophy.

Finally, how can the industry remove more hurdles to empower the development and adoption of digital healthcare? More data at faster flow rates with higher data integrity accelerate the improvement of AI technologies. But data security and individual privacy remain top priorities in healthcare, which inevitably slow progress. Are we going to sacrifice privacy for better care? Research studies have shown that the millennials are more willing to give up their health data in exchange for a cheaper insurance rate. Millennials are more comfortable with the fact that Google and Facebook may know their health conditions better than their doctors do.

In summary, it is beyond our imagination today how big data and AI technologies will transform healthcare in just a generation or two, and I truly believe that technology is the ultimate solution to bring equal and affordable healthcare to everyone. This book will not only open your mind to the possibilities that exist at the intersection of healthcare and data, but it will also inspire more people to embark on this exciting journey.

REFERENCES

1. CMS.gov. (2019). *National health expenditure accounts.* Retrieved from: https://www.cms.gov/Research-Statistics-Data-and-Systems/Statistics-Trends-and-Reports/NationalHealthExpendData/NationalHealthAccountsHistorical.html
2. CMS.gov. (2018). *National health expenditure projections 2017–2026 Forecast summary.* Retrieved from: https://www.cms.gov/Research-Statistics-Data-and-Systems/Statistics-Trends-and-Reports/NationalHealthExpendData/Downloads/ForecastSummary.pdf
3. FDA website. (2019). *Digital health.* Retrieved from: https://www.fda.gov/MedicalDevices/DigitalHealth/default.htm
4. Atherton, J. (2011). Development of the electronic health record. *AMA Journal of Ethics*, *13*(3), 186–189.
5. HealthIT.gov. (2019). *Regional extension centers.* Retrieved from: https://www.healthit.gov/topic/regional-extension-centers-recs

6. Wikipedia. (2019). *Health insurance portability and accountability act.* Retrieved from https://en.wikipedia.org/wiki/Health_Insurance_Portability_and_Accountability_Act

7. Startup Health. (2018). *Top trends in digital health funding.* Retrieved from https://healthtransformer.co/top-trends-in-digital-health-funding-from-startup-healths-mid-year-report-d6c1749b5df8

8. Rijmenam, M. (2015). *A short history of big data.* Retrieved from https://datafloq.com/read/big-data-history/239

9. Fleming, N. (2018). How artificial intelligence is changing drug development. *Nature, 557*, S55–57

10. Smith, S. (2018). *101 Startups using AI in drug discovery.* Retrieved from https://blog.benchsci.com/startups-using-artificial-intelligence-in-drug-discovery

11. CB Insights Report. (2016). *64 Healthcare IoT startups in patient monitoring, clinical efficiency, biometrics and more.* Retrieved from https://www.cbinsights.com/research/iot-healthcare-market-map-company-list/

12. United Health Motion Program. (2019). *United health motion program.* Retrieved from https://www.uhc.com/employer/programs-tools/for-employees/unitedhealthcare-motion

13. Maddox, T. (2014). *TechRepublic. Wearables have a dirty little secret: 50% of users lose interest.* Retrieved from https://www.techrepublic.com/article/wearables-have-a-dirty-little-secret-most-people-lose-interest/

14. FDA press release.(2018). *FDA permits marketing of artificial intelligence-based device to detect certain diabetes-related eye problems.* Retrieved from https://www.fda.gov/newsevents/newsroom/pressannouncements/ucm604357.htm

15. Dar, P. (2018). *Google's machine learning model can detect cancer in real-time.* Retrieved from https://www.analyticsvidhya.com/blog/2018/04/googles-machine-learning-model-can-detect-cancer-real-time/

16. Lardieri, A. (2018). AI beats doctors at cancer diagnosis. *US News.* Retrieved from https://www.usnews.com/news/health-care-news/articles/2018-05-28/artificial-intelligence-beats-dermatologists-at-diagnosing-skin-cancer

17. Editorial (2018). AI diagnostics need attention. *Nature, 555*, 285–286

18. Wikipedia. (2019). *Watson (computer).* Retrieved from https://en.wikipedia.org/wiki/Watson_(computer)

19. Galeon, D. (2016). *IBM's Watson AI recommends same treatment as doctors in 99% of cancer cases.* Retrieved from https://futurism.com/ibms-watson-ai-recommends-same-treatment-as-doctors-in-99-of-cancer-cases

20. Chen, A. (2018). *IBM's Watson game unsafe recommendations for treating cancer.* Retrieved from https://www.theverge.com/2018/7/26/17619382/ibms-watson-cancer-ai-healthcare-science

21. National Association of Chronic Disease Directors. (2019). *Why we need public health to improve healthcare.* Retrieved from https://www.chronicdisease.org/page/whyweneedph2imphc

22. Editorial team. (2017). *Artificial intelligence and the move towards preventive healthcare.* Retrieved from https://insidebigdata.com/2017/12/13/artificial-intelligence-move-towards-preventive-healthcare/

23. Zhegin, P. (2017). The role of AI in the future of healthcare. *Venture Beat.* Retrieved from https://venturebeat.com/2017/07/19/the-role-of-ai-in-the-future-of-health-care/

CHAPTER 2

THE EVOLVING INTERNET OF THINGS (IOT) IN HEALTHCARE

The Impact of IoT and Communication Technology on Health Care Services

Jerry Power, Steve Garske, and Ken Hayashida

INTRODUCTION

The healthcare industry is in a technological crossroad where innovation in digital communication intersects with emerging Internet-of-Things (IoT) technology. This nexus is changing the relationships between patients, healthcare care providers, health care systems, and governments. Advancements in consumer digital and communications technology causes doctors, hospitals, and health systems to evaluate the impact of these rapidly evolving technologies in the context of the complex healthcare administrative, regulatory, and clinical requirements.

The world of technology continues to benefit from miniaturized form-factors, such as, improving accuracy, growing functionality, and accelerating speed. Meanwhile, the administrative and operational requirements in the healthcare space are complex, multi-faceted, and shaped by regulatory oversight. This chapter considers the impact of advancing digital communication technology on the

Transforming Healthcare with Big Data and AI, pages 21–41.
Copyright © 2020 by Information Age Publishing
21

delivery of healthcare services by individual healthcare providers and organizational healthcare systems.

TODAY'S HEALTHCARE IOT

Standard business practices in the communications industry has resulted in mass-marketing of increasingly powerful computational and communication devices such as touch screen-enabled phones and tablets. Developers of various health-related devices and software are building on these technologies to market these wellness products and applications as "intelligent" or "smart." Evaluation of these health-monitoring tools and wearable devices is in progress in many clinical settings. While consumer-grade devices have the potential to increase the quantity of data collected from an individual, some clinicians question the accuracy and clinical validity of data collected by consumer devices. There is the clinical risk of erroneous medical decisions based upon inaccurate health data measurements from consumer devices. There are also behavioral and cultural issues which could introduce error in measurement outside of the controlled setting in a clinical medical environment.

There are many clinical studies evaluating the use of consumer fitness devices in patients with specific chronic diseases. These publications allow for the controlled observation of device use by medical researchers. Evaluation of the accuracy of these consumer devices to prognosticate clinical outcome or benefit to the patient requires long-term, multi-center, and multi-year longitudinal analyses. Clinical research of patients with specific medical diagnoses or conditions requires clinical validation studies. Without these validation studies, healthcare practitioners will have difficulty prognosticating outcome based upon specific consumer-grade devices. Until such longitudinal clinical outcome studies are concluded, the clinical management protocols will retain existing clinical guidelines and recommendations.

In addition to the clinical and scientific questions, administrative and operational requirements exist for medical groups and hospitals. Healthcare systems and medical centers maintain internal procedures and policies which define clinical work flows. These clinical procedures require a protocol for communication between medical staff and personnel in order to efficiently move patients through facilities. Internal regulations and medical center policies reflect prior experience and events. Sometimes these procedures have been based upon legacy paper and pen processes.

Healthcare system and medical center policies do not normally contemplate integration of information flow from environments outside the traditional hospital or medical office examination room. Security, privacy, and regulatory compliance measures impact these communication protocols and information flow into and within medical centers, medical groups, and between care providers. Security and privacy risks are addressed by administrative policies and review of procedures, but emerging threats continue to require attention of hospital administrators and all staff.

Therefore, reception of the information from consumer health and medical devices by the health care system will require insight to care provider work flow and the corporate responsibilities internal to the healthcare operation. Integration of consumer devices into clinical communication workflows requires a dedicated investment of time and resources that may be outside the existing budget for many medical institutions and systems.

Meanwhile, digital networks interconnecting communication devices grow in speed and reliability with decreasing cost to consumers. Reference databases, artificial intelligence, man-machine interface systems (MMI), and cloud services are adding utility and capability to these proliferating and pervasive networks. When applied to the healthcare field, the combination of smart device and instantaneous digital networking suggests a future where individual patients can communicate medical and health related information on a 24–7 basis with healthcare providers. This optimistically presents a future where the health care system, specific medical facilities, and care providers can show improved outcomes for challenging patient populations. Further, people living in geographic areas where specific medical care services may be limited or inaccessible will be able to communicate accurate medical data more quickly and efficiently.

Progress in communication technology is already impacting the delivery of healthcare services today with concomitant expenses and risks. Improved communications have the potential to further improve healthcare efficiencies, but they also increase the need to safeguard protected health information, ensure data integrity and security, and adhere to new regulatory regulations.

These technology-enabled improvements may appear if healthcare providers rethink their current perceptions of the healthcare industry. The understanding of outcomes and metrics are shifting from facility and provider-based measures to patient-centric measures that require a much larger ecosystem of participating partners. The idea of a hospital as an isolated institution transforms to a community-centric ecosystem of care delivery and management. As a technology, IoT will play a critical role in this transition, but other technologies and factors must also play a role. The cultural change in the definition of healthcare across a community will occur as community-wide networks develop and information management matures. Ultimately healthcare becomes less about tactically managing one illness and more about strategically managing communities to gain a larger vision of wellness across the populations served.

This forward-looking view of healthcare as an efficient, community centric, participatory ecosystem is transformative. This vision will evolve over time enabled by technology and implemented over a series of digital transformation projects. Ultimately, many such digital transformation projects are required and the order and speed at which they are pursued will vary widely as each community seeks to optimize the evolutionary process to meet local needs.

This should not be taken to imply that the application of these advanced technologies is ready for mass market deployment, but evidence suggests that healthcare institutions across the world are deploying and testing components of critical elements necessary to allow the healthcare industry to take the next step.

CHALLENGES IN THE HEALTHCARE IMPLEMENTATION OF IOT DEVICES

While the capabilities of these cutting-edge technology systems are truly inspiring and offers the potential to improve healthcare outcomes while reducing systemic costs, technology should be understood as a tool. How these tools are applied by institutions and agencies determine the outcomes to be realized.

Healthcare institutions are built utilizing equipment from a variety of suppliers and thus maintenance of this complicated system must occur in a multi-vendor environment. While an individual vendor can achieve wonders with technology, there are different challenges when introducing that same technology in an environment supporting a combination of pre-existing vendors with unique configurations and customized deployments. Implementation of prior packages and deployments can be customized for healthcare environments. Typically, this mix of vendors are in competition with each other, often leaving the healthcare IT teams in the middle. Moreover, once the system is installed and certified for operations, the healthcare IT staff may face demands from medical staff to continue to support legacy implementations. Therefore, healthcare IT staff are faced with an effort to maintain a complex, multi-vendor infrastructure that is unique to their institution.

Data security is increasingly in the news as "mischief makers" seek to gain access to network structures that are intended to be secure. These threats are often carried out for bragging rights and sometime for the sinister purpose of causing harm. While healthcare institutions act to detect and thwart such behavior, it is impossible to prevent every possible misbehavior. Complicating matters further, some of these activities are simply the result of human, but well-intentioned, error.

Tangentially related to these data security issues are data privacy issues. Security ensures that health data is properly protected from external parties. Privacy relates to assurances that data use is limited to the purposes intended by the patient. Patients generally trust their doctor and want to provide their doctor with the best information possible in order to ensure the highest level of healthcare. This does not suggest that same level of trust applies to the system administrators or the support structures that assist the doctor. Patients want to have an active voice in determining when and how their healthcare data is utilized by the larger healthcare community.

The healthcare environment is fluid. Patients change doctors, see specialists, change insurance carriers, visit multiple clinics, and move between hospitals and medical centers. Doctors change hospital affiliations, alter partnerships, and change insurance company relationships. The healthcare system is structured with the expectation that the logical linkages within the healthcare ecosystem will evolve over time. In a data-centric world this fluidity forces data within the ecosystem to also move. As new devices and capabilities appear, these new sources of data must be integrated with historic records.

Technology, particularly when it is first introduced, is expensive to develop, deploy, train, and build processes. It often obsoletes existing equipment or forces expensive upgrade procedures onto legacy systems needed to maintain system-level compatibility. These management and administrative challenges are compounded by the pace of regulatory change and by tightening budgets due to decreases in reimbursement for services. The aging population curve in the United States increases demand for higher acuity medical services as health care administrators are being requested to reduce costs, make more efficient use of bed capacity, and optimize staffing levels.

A STACK OF ENGINEERING PROGRESS FOR IOT IMPLEMENTATION IN HEALTHCARE

Technology can be considered as a tool enabling new information services and approaches to delivery of healthcare while disrupting slower and less responsive processes. The information superhighway carrying medical information should be engineered with specific routing of traffic, rights of priority in traffic lanes, and assured velocities of travel. Continued improvements in efficiency is becoming more challenging and complex to implement. Generally speaking, the health care professions have automated most of the legacy processes that could be automated. Additional technical advancement needs to be coupled with procedural and process innovation.

Innovation in the engineering of digital networking and communications devices continues to improve speed, decrease power consumption, shrink microprocessor chip sets, and increase memory storage capacity. A stack of technological effects relevant to healthcare can be described.

1. **IoT Device Physical Factors:** The semiconductor and device industry continues to reduce the size and power footprint of IoT devices. This serves to reduce the cost of the devices while simultaneously increasing the amount of data produced. In the healthcare space this leads to improving performance, accuracy of measurement, and sensor diversity for the patient and provider to consider. The global emergence of these health and medical devices continues at a brisk pace that was not possible in prior generations. As use of consumer-level health tracking and fitness devices grows, health care applications will appear with reduced latency, lower costs, greater quantities of data, and growing reliability in obtaining accurate and automatic physiologic measurements.

2. **Network Communication Velocity and Bandwidth:** Wi-fi, LTE, and 5G wireless networking topologies offer increasing digital bandwidth available to host mobile communication devices. When applied to medi-

cal communications, users can move over larger ranges of distance, geographies and environments while maintaining real-time digital communication at higher velocities.

3. **Data Warehousing and Analytics:** The recording of large amounts of health and wellness observations requires warehousing of these health data in centralized databases. Advancements in data warehouse services and analytics are improving the experience of building, operating, and maintaining large quantities of secure health and medical information for research and reference purposes. University-level affiliated medical centers and commercial healthcare organizations routinely utilize these systems for research purposes.

4. **Patient Transport Process:** Currently, the transport of patients to a healthcare facility and provider for medical assessment is the norm. However, personal health and medical information could be collected from medical-grade consumer devices and presented to the healthcare team prior to transporting the patient. More accurate and efficient routing of emergency cases to match the patient's needs with the facility's services is one potentiality. Efficiencies can also be realized by freeing the practice of healthcare from inventories of specialized medical equipment that are tied to a specific location and pushing lower cost devices to lower acuity levels of care.

5. **Local and Global Intelligence:** A wealth of insight will soon become available to support individual and community-level care decision making. The application of machine learning and artificial intelligence processes to extremely large datasets may reveal relationships in community-level, population-wide datasets that individual healthcare practitioners would be unable to observe by themselves. Progress is being made in the automation of data analysis, machine-learning, and artificial Intelligence (AI) to transform voluminous data into actionable metrics. As wireless networks proliferate, previously underserved populations will have easier access to medical knowledge and health education content. At a physical level, this data will allow more accurate and timely communication with individual users as they take advantage of new mobility services for access to care. Healthcare services will have mobility rather than being fixed to specific offices or locations.

OBJECTIVES IN APPLYING THE INTERNET OF THINGS TO HEALTH CARE SERVICES AND DELIVERY

As the effects of these interactive technological innovations build, objectives in application of the technology to health care services must be considered. As a general observation, it is expected that IoT and technology in general may enable gains in the healthcare industry by addressing one or more of the following objectives:

1. **Identification of Health Trends and Medical Needs for the Individual User:** Communication technology will assist in identifying individuals with changes to physical function and, perhaps, the need for medical assistance, support, and care. Technology can also assist defining the types of health care services required in terms of urgency, procedure type, and the location for that care. Advancements in technology, when applied in healthcare, will continue the shift to a predictive and preventive model by empowering individual patients, care providers, and health systems with population wide insight.

2. **Matching the Individual to Health System Service Resources:** Technology will improve communication between healthcare resources and individuals with the need for assistance, support, and care. Once identified, users can locate and communicate with networks of healthcare professionals with a wide range of healthcare affiliated resources, including sub-specialists, primary care, pharmacies, nursing care, transportation services, social workers, community resources, and caregivers.

3. **Monitoring of Community and Population-wide Health Metrics and Analysis:** Advances in technology will improve preventive health care services provided on a community-wide level. Moreover, progress in the personalization of healthcare delivery cannot be achieved without equal progress on a community and population-wide basis.

4. **Monitoring of Efficient Use and Quality of Health Care Services:** Healthcare institution improve the efficiency and quality of care services. Technology can be utilized to drive these efficiencies to a larger stage by use of data services to interoperate between health care centers and systems. For example, this same technology could be used to link segmented hospitals and trauma centers into a unified, regional healthcare network.

5. **Personalization of Community Environmental Metrics:** It has been widely accepted that health issues are often driven by the environment. But healthcare institutions do not, as a matter of course, collect environmental data in the community to assess how patients live their lives and include that data as part of health records. If the healthcare professional had information focused on individual environments, personalized treatment plans can include recommendations tailored to environmental factors impacting patient well-being.

EXAMPLES OF NEXT-GENERATION IOT INTEGRATION IMPACTING HEALTHCARE

Next-generation, health care systems will be based on platform architectures that clearly segment the infrastructure, applications, devices, and communications systems into different logical layers. The following examples describe a cross section of evolutionary programs that illustrate efforts to create forward looking systems that meet current needs while simultaneously providing a path for forward growth.

Examples of Identification of Health Trends and Medical Needs for the Individual User

Some IoT devices require patients to self-monitor and self-manage their health while at home. The simple fact that a part of the population is motivated to participate in the healthcare process is a positive step forward for healthcare in general; however, the home health technology environment is not always HIPPA compliant. This should raise questions about data authenticity, quality, and privacy as this data passes through a gateway into a HIPPA compliant domain. Additionally, the home-health care device market often does not receive FDA approval, which means the data from these devices are not calibrated or tested against an industry standard; the same data from different devices might be calibrated or measured differently making the reported data (and healthcare integration efforts) vendor dependent.

In another example of physiologic observation of individual users, a team of researchers from the Massachusetts Institute of Technology in Cambridge created RF-Pose, a wireless smart-home system that employs artificial intelligence to sense people's movements through walls [1]. The development team utilized a neural network to analyze how radio signals bounce off people's bodies — even when they're on the opposite side of a wall. During a recent research study, the neural network was able to successfully extrapolate these findings to sense a subject's postures and movements. The researchers are using this sensor technology, coupled with AI intelligence, to work with physicians to allow physicians to monitor patients with conditions like Parkinson's Disease or Multiple Sclerosis. The goal is to assist the physicians understanding of the disease progression, without requiring a patient to wear personal sensors. Dina Katabi, team leader and professor in MIT's Computer Science and Artificial Intelligence Laboratory reported, "We've seen that monitoring patients' walking speed and ability to do basic activities on their own gives healthcare providers a window into their lives that they didn't have before, which could be meaningful for a whole range of diseases." The researchers intend to implement a consent mechanism for RF-Pose before deploying other "real-world" applications as well. These mechanisms require the participant to simply perform a specific set of movements prior to the system monitoring the environment to obtain a baseline set of data on which to compare the ongoing surveillance by the AI system.

Northwestern Medicine, a Chicago based health care system, is launching an artificial intelligence center focused on cardiovascular disease with funding from a $25 million charitable donation [2]. The Bluhm Family Charitable Foundation's gift builds on the foundation's previous financial donations to Northwestern Medicine. In 2005, the foundation — formed by Chicago philanthropist and real estate developer Neil G. Bluhm — established the Northwestern Medicine Bluhm

Cardiovascular Institute. The new gift will support the investigation into how advancements in artificial intelligence and machine learning can help improve cardiovascular disease diagnosis, treatment, and research. According to Patrick M. McCarthy, MD, executive director of the cardiovascular institute, "Artificial intelligence is the next frontier in breakthrough medicine, and Northwestern Medicine is leading the way by incorporating this emerging technology throughout its cardiovascular programs."

Medtronic created an application-based diabetes management assistant, called Sugar.iQ [3]. The Sugar.IQ application, which is now available to users of Medtronic's Guardian Connect continuous glucose monitoring system via Apple's App Store, employs artificial intelligence and analytics from IBM Watson Health to analyze how certain foods, insulin dosages and daily routines influence glucose levels. The Medtronic and IBM Watson Health's goal for the application is to provide patients with personalized guidance addressing how best to control their glucose levels. Patients who used the Sugar.IQ app spent 36 more minutes per day in the healthy glucose range than they did prior to downloading the application, according to research presented at the 78th Scientific Sessions of the American Diabetes Association.

A research team from the University of Waterloo in Ontario, Canada, is developing a new method to detect changes in diabetes patients' glucose levels without the need for an invasive blood draw [4]. Traditionally, diabetes patients must monitor their blood glucose levels by drawing blood via a finger prick several times a day. To avoid the need for frequent blood draws, the researchers are working with Google and the German hardware company Infineon to utilize radar and artificial intelligence technologies to detect changes in patients' blood glucose levels. Initial tests indicate these technologies were 85 percent as accurate as traditional blood analysis. The project employs radar to send high-frequency radio waves into a patient's blood sample and the returned radio waves contain information about the patient's glucose levels. Researchers proceed to analyze this information with AI algorithms that detect glucose changes based on 500-plus wave characteristics, such as how long the radio waves take to "bounce back" to the device sensor.

George Shaker, PhD, an adjunct assistant professor of electrical and computer engineering at the University of Waterloo and leader of the research team, envisions a day when there will be the ability to analyze blood conditions inside the body without actually having to sample any fluid. Continued research efforts are expected to improve sensor sensitivity and ultimately allow these advanced detectors to obtain results through a patient's skin. In the future, it may be possible to build the technology into a smartwatch type device to actively monitor a patient's health in hospital quality data.

*Examples of Matching of Individual Needs to Health System
Service Resources*

An example of communication technology intersecting with medical devices occurs daily when paramedics utilize digital communication technologies to share medical data from devices in the field with supporting emergency rooms during emergency response. This allows the first-responders to provide rapid diagnostics and immediate medical interventions in the field or during patient transport. Additionally, medical personnel in the ER can be notified of the pending arrival of a patient in distress and prepare emergency care resources prior to arrival of the patient. This same concept can also be employed to permit individuals to send personal healthcare information to their doctor before less acute needs arise.

For several years, there have been publications of specific use cases when digital communication technology is applied to post-operative monitoring of patients upon discharge from the hospital. This monitoring of patient out-comes is helpful to address government mandated metrics reported by hospitals to regulators.

Geisinger's Steele Institute for Healthcare Innovation is deploying an artificial intelligence tool at Geisinger Medical Center in Danville [5]. The AI tool, which Jvion brands as its "cognitive clinical success machine" solution, will aid Geisinger Medical Center in reducing avoidable readmissions related to chronic obstructive pulmonary disease, a group of lung diseases by using patient-care data to identify early warning indicators that can trigger action before the situation becomes critical.

*Examples of Monitoring of Community and Population-Wide
Health Metrics and Analysis*

An example of community-wide healthcare technology being used to help monitor risk for future disease is the monitoring of vaccination rates in California schools. State-mandated reporting of the immunization status of children was previously handled by way of primary care physicians completing hand-signed paper-based forms. Previously, these manually completed forms conveyed dates of each vaccine for each pupil. However, processing of these forms by primary care offices, school district personnel, and school nurses was manual and time-consuming. Development of digital vaccine registries and district-wide, student health databases and applications permit sharing of data with district-wide analysis across the population of students in each school site in a community.

Previously published clinical research on "herd-immunity" defines the vaccination-rates required in a community to protect children from vaccine-preventable infectious disease. Therefore, the population-specific data which is calculable from school district-based student health metrics provides an assessment of the risk of contagion and spread of vaccine preventable infectious disease in schools.

Compliance by healthcare providers in a community with public health recommendations is visible on a geographic basis. These metrics can also provide temporal insight to characterize the effect of public health messages on vulnerable populations. Expansion of these capabilities will make use of metrics to reveal issues impacting delivery of care, including the alignment and implementation of regional public health recommendations by community-level health care providers. Advancement in the communication technology will allow revision of these recommendations on a timelier basis.

Examples of Monitoring of Efficiencies within and the Quality of Health Care Services

Healthcare professionals have constraints on their time spent per patient encounter. Consider an 8-hour work shift, not including required break time with a ratio of 1 nurse to 8 patients. This leaves the nurse 60 minutes to care for one patient per 8-hour shift. This does not include the time to interface with digital documentation systems. Assuming the nurse logs in and reviews existing health care records for the first 10 minutes of the patient intake process and then spends 20 minutes at the end of each patient visit updating the records, a mere 30 minutes is left to interact with the patient. As IoT increases the amount of data in the records, the amount of time required for records review will increase and face-to-face patient time will logically decrease.

One challenge facing IoT deployments relates to the need that IoT data be self-organizing. The increased volumes of data cannot be allowed to reduce doctor-patient time and should be targeted to increasing patient time compared to today's current practice. To do this, as IoT devices generate patient specific data, the data must be automatically logged into the patient's medical record to minimize the human time required for data management. Further, the patient's record must be self-organizing (based on AI) so the most important data is prioritized in presentation to medical staff. Perhaps the default setting should be that patient records are presented to the medical staff in terms of priority with the most critical points being presented ahead of lower priority data.

Fortunately, several of the top EHR vendors are nearing the release of IoT based AI systems that will assist clinicians with the basic input of data. A major complaint by physicians and care givers is the increased time to complete the electronic record, and decreased time with the patient and their family. By restructuring a patient visit and utilizing IoT and AI, many aspects of this challenge can be overcome. At least one EHR vendor has a prototype of this patient visit workflow redesign. It consists of various IoT devices that gather information prior to the visit, then uploads this to the patients EHR at the time of the visit. Once the doctor walks into the patient room, two video and audio arrays monitor and track the conversation and exam. The EHR is populated with the IoT device information, as well as the conversation and exam. Medications, orders, diagnosis, and many other elements are populated in the EHR prior to and during the visit. This saves clinicians both time and effort.

A group of researchers from the Center for Robotic Simulation and Education at the Los Angeles-based Keck School of Medicine at the University of Southern California have implemented artificial intelligence to measure surgeons' performance and described their experiences in an article for JAMA Surgery [6]. The current standard for evaluating surgeons is peer review by an expert evaluator, either during surgery or from video footage following the procedure. To improve the accuracy of the process and decrease the need for expert evaluators, the researchers developed a method to automatically analyze data captured by surgical robots. Robots represent high end IoT devices that can feed data to AI based learning systems to analyze performance and then actively learn from the process. The researchers employed a Da Vinci System to collect performance metrics and then used AI algorithms to recognize patterns in a surgeons' performance. They found the algorithms could "objectively measure surgeon performance and anticipate patient outcomes." "Systems data captured directly from the robot provide an opportunity to more accurately and objectively measure surgeon performance." Similar types of technology are expected to be applicable to support personalized surgeon training as well.

Efficient use of health care space is also helped by the development of algorithms that are capable of monitoring the duration of time required to complete procedures. A more precise understanding of process timing allows equipment inventory to efficiently manage sterilization procedures, decrease idle time in key areas, and improve the ability of support staff to prepare equipment and rooms for subsequent use.

Innovation in the use of digital communication devices impacts how medical care is rendered. The growth of telemedicine services across the United States over the past twenty years has helped to address access to care issues in rural communities. These same technologies also assist urban medical centers when consulting with specialty physicians who may be on-call for multiple centers. These panels assist in situations requiring higher levels of medical expertise to diagnose and treat patients with complex illnesses. The communication network becomes a force multiplier for the region.

In many medical centers across the nation, radiologists remotely review and report results of radiographic procedures. Electrocardiograms (EKG's), Echocardiograms, and some radiographic procedures (x-rays, CT scans, and MRI scans) are examples of medical procedures which can be ordered on an emergency basis from a major hospital ER and where the review of the results can be reported by physicians that are distant to the immediate site of care. The ability to gain immediate and mobile access to rich, high-definition video content by these licensees may significantly impact their quality of work, care, and life.

There are some medical centers where "on-call" radiologists are available in very distant locations, including outside the borders of the United States. This allows night-time emergency procedures to be reviewed by physicians working a day shift in another time zone. This time shifting of work is relevant to the accuracy and speed of reporting and in the well-being of physician specialists and the patients served.

In another example of digital technology helping to address efficiencies in patient care, the "eICU" project at Emory University's medical center built the ability to supplement on-site critical care medical personnel with similar personnel situated in a communications center on the opposite side of the world. By building this "eICU" capability, night-shift management of patients in Atlanta is assisted by day-shift critical care physicians in Perth, Australia. This is an example of how medical device data can be shared through a digital network to improve the well-being of patients while improving efficiencies in the healthcare workforce.

Example of Personalization of Community Environmental Metrics

In 2012, the Air Louisville project partnered local funders, the city of Louisville, and Propeller Health to deploy 300 asthma inhaler sensors that track administration of each use of asthma medication from the inhaler. Scaling of the program to over 1000 sensors and patients was funded by the Robert Woods Johnson Foundation. This program aligned these new devices with public health interests in controlling asthma on the municipal level. Although the project did not personalize environmental air-quality measurement, it did personalize the monitoring and tracking of asthma inhaler use and asthma intervention. Heat mapping generated by inhaler use data illustrated areas of higher inhaler use while different mapped regions correlated to higher hospitalization rates, suggesting that higher incidence of hospitalizations for asthma occur in areas of less compliance with asthma interventions. This complex project involves calibration of sensor data to maps and other environmental data from the city of Louisville. The project can be reviewed at www.airlouisville.com.

TECHNOLOGY ENABLED CAPABILITIES AND ISSUES

Calibration, testing, and tracking of home-healthcare devices is expensive and drives the price of many home-health care tools outside the reach of many consumers. As an alternative, given that the ability to process data is increasing at such a rapid rate, information reported by a specific class of medical devices might be aligned to an industry standard protocol. Several candidate protocols currently exist.

The effort required to organize data to draw a medical technician's attention to the most important information can be a simple or complicated process. Some organizational rules in healthcare are standardized through medical training. For example, the heart rate, temperature, and blood pressure are universally recorded and should be reported as one of the first records of any electronic healthcare record. Many of the current EHRs allow for the customization of the record now, with new decision support algorithms also being created regularly.

Other indicators are more nuanced, and their priority depends upon other data records. By analogy, over-the-horizon early-warning systems deployed by defense agencies quantify risk of attack by utilizing radar. In those monitoring systems, the impending danger is determined based on the existence of a complex set of trigger warnings. If conditions in a trigger situation are met, an alert or automated response is transmitted to an appropriate authority. In the case of medical care, physiologists and physicians are aware that specific physiologic measurements are a potential indicator of concern warranting closer evaluation. Those conditions cause the monitoring process to message warnings. Different medical specialties may be characterized differently in the expert system, allowing a specific doctor to have their issues uniquely flagged. Moreover, one doctor will be able to observe the issues that have been raised to other doctors, thereby improving doctor-to-doctor coordination.

In the United States, the majority of the healthcare needs are supported by insurance companies and overseen by regulators. Most patients are supportive of any advances in healthcare that improve the level of healthcare or reduce the cost of services, however, there is significant concern that the same data that allows improvement in the diagnostic/treatment processes will be employed by insurance companies to identify higher risk individuals to influence coverage decisions or alter monthly premiums. Despite promises from the insurers this will not occur, consumers are wary that the potential exists. The existence of a promise from an untrusted financial stakeholder with profit incentives are not comforting. Regulators have been positioned to serve as a check and balance against the insurance industry, but regulators move slowly compared to ever-evolving technologies.

Economics represents another issue facing the industry. The cost of deploying IoT systems in a sufficient density to create a sufficiently significant blanket of data is staggering. Making use of incentives would shift some of the burden of creating this 'fabric' of IoT devices from the healthcare institutions to the public. For example, if healthcare providers gather environmental data from privately deployed IoT devices, it means the healthcare industry does not need to duplicate that investment with industry owned IoT devices. Incentives can increase deployment in areas with economic means, but targeting specific areas would allow costs to be targeted yet will also contribute to a growing medical data divide where those with the economic means will have better healthcare than others. Ultimately insurance companies and/or government agencies must play an increased role in deploying these IoT systems to ensure the data coverage (and data driven healthcare in general) is not rationed.

The described concerns are problematic in today's healthcare environment and addressing these concerns may improve healthcare efficiencies in the near term. However, longer term, as these kinds of monitoring devices become pervasive, these issues will grow in magnitude and solutions will become harder to adopt. After all, it is easier to repair a plane while it is on the ground compared to in flight.

As IoT systems are expanded, the volume of data produced by the IoT devices will grow exponentially. The real-time nature of the data allows response time improvements and also improve the ability to predict future health issues. However, predictions rely on historic data which implies a need to retain these vast volumes of real-time data as legacy records that can be incorporated into predictive analytics. The growing volume of IoT devices and the increased need for retention of historic data creates an expanding data management problem. There are alternative proposals that suggest placing intelligence at the edge of a network to filter the data thereby reducing the amount of data managed centrally. However, inherent in such proposals is the implication that the need for data is well understood. While reducing the data volume at the edge saves on storage and communication cost, it also reduces the amount of data that can drive predictive health care analytics. In many ways, data is like an investment and filtering data at the edge may save costs near term but also reduces the potential that can be derived from the data. Given that network communications and data storage costs continue to plummet, the tipping point that determines whether data should be saved or discarded will continue to shift from filter-based proposals toward centralized data repositories.

Centralization or decentralization of data represents another area of potential activity. Centralized repositories have been the industry norm for approaching data management issues. While distributed database systems have been in existence for many years, the appearance of blockchain as a community managed alternative to the centralized system have drawn increased interest. It is difficult to discuss blockchain systems as a whole because there are so many incompatible variations of blockchain making it a challenge to compare data management alternatives. In general, blockchain was developed as a means of conducting data transfers in an environment where there is no trusted central authority. In blockchain, a community agrees to work together to support a shared data repository. The coordination required between the involved carries the baggage of reduced performance. But this overhead allows improved privacy and security if a central authority cannot be trusted. What is unclear is whether blockchain eliminates the need for a trusted relationship, whether it fills an operational need until a trusted relationship can be built, or whether the performance penalty that comes with current blockchain systems melts away as communications costs continue to fall.

Environment data, such as weather data, includes data such as pollen counts. This data is typically created from digital models rather than actual sensor readings. While this data is useful, it lacks the clinical significance of data that is generated from a network of local sensors. Some state and local agencies have deployed sensors that measure ozone, carbon monoxide, nitrogen dioxide, and sulfur dioxide (components of smog) for research purposes in limited areas. Real-time data from these systems is utilized by some commercial organizations (e.g. purpleair.com, airbeam) as low accuracy data streams. While these systems provide real-time data, the nature of the data collection methodology is often not well documented which limits the usefulness of the data in a healthcare setting. For example, some of these systems fail to distinguish indoor from outdoor air quality or clearly identify mobile from fixed-site data collection. Moreover, the accuracy of air-quality sensors is sometimes related to the quality of the detection sensors, but the specifications of the specific sensors are often not disclosed. Organizations such as The South Coast Air Quality Management District looks at these early systems as a first step and is continuing their efforts to build and expand on the capabilities and assessments.

To date, there have been many proposals that suggest that Machine Learning and AI algorithms can be directly applied to assist emergency services personnel during times of crisis; these same systems can be made available to citizens for improved information access while emergency services are en-route. The capabilities of these AI driven systems are proportional to the amount of data available to them. While the capabilities of these systems are already impressive, the data ingested to date is largely professional quality data which implies they could be doing demonstrably more if they were able to tap the full extent of the digital world.

In a note of caution, researchers at the Massachusetts Institute of Technology in Boston created what they've dubbed the "world's first psychopath AI" [7]. The artificial intelligence algorithm, nicknamed "Norman" after the character Norman Bates in Alfred Hitchcock's film "Psycho," generates captions for Rorschach-style inkblot psychological tests. Because the researchers trained the algorithm on violent content from what they call "the darkest corners of Reddit," Norman applied more disturbing descriptions than industry standard image captioning models. In one example, a standard image captioning model described an inkblot as "a group of birds sitting on top of a tree branch." However, Norman provided the caption "a man is electrocuted and catches to death." The researchers stressed their reason for developing Norman was to underscore a foundational principle of AI — use of AI to achieve better treatment of mental disorders is highly dependent on the data that drive the AI engine. The MIT research further demonstrated that data employed to teach a machine learning algorithm can significantly influence its future behavior. This also suggested that some mental disorders can be exacerbated by exposure to biased data and perhaps a possible treatment might be influenced by altering the prevailing data.

THE ROAD FORWARD

There is a consensus understanding that increased volumes of data can improve healthcare outcomes while also lowering costs. However, the operational structures that evolved to ensure health care quality cannot be extended to cover all the data that might have a positive impact on healthcare outcomes. The current trend is to ask consumers to contribute their generated data into an ecosystem managed by the healthcare and insurance industry. Unfortunately, this evolutionary push will be impeded by consumer trust issues given that the healthcare industry is overseen by insurance and various governmental agencies.

Further complicating this issue is the fact that the healthcare industry, including hospitals, medical centers, pharmacies, and third-party medical management companies) do not have the staff or insight into the dramatic expansion coming to reality in data and communication technologies (big data, artificial intelligence, Internet-of-Things, and more). Delegating or outsourcing efforts to manage the growing number of data driven healthcare processes to external services has limits unless these outsource service companies are willing to assume liability for automated healthcare decision making processes.

A new path forward is necessary to support a healthcare system that is able to incorporate all data that might serve to improve healthcare outcomes. Patients will not be satisfied releasing their personal data to a managed healthcare ecosystem unless they are provided direct involvement in the use of their data. Personal involvement in data decision making implies patients may also wish to make that same data available to parties outside the traditional healthcare ecosystem. Data is data and it does not become healthcare data until it is put into a managed data infrastructure; that same data can be processed for purposes outside the HIPPA managed bubble with the user being directly involved in the process. It is possible that a manager of these data structures can refuse to accept data from devices which they consider to be unacceptable. Device manufacturers may seek to have their devices certified by one or more of these ecosystem managers. Data infrastructure managers, data producing devices, and healthcare applications can exist outside the managed environment to provide guidance for external patient advice portals. These external systems can be bound by geography, insurance coverage, or political designations. Effectively there are multiple healthcare ecosystems, some with industry/government oversight and control while others do not. Both the regulated and unregulated environments should be accessible to the greater medical community, with researchers and public health personnel, possibly having access to all of the data.

It is possible that the role of a primary care physician in the near-future will begin to shift from that of hands-on care at a designated office appointment to a personal healthcare advisor. Perhaps, as part of a future appointment process, patients may interact with one or more healthcare services driven by artificial intelligence and machine learning logic. This may accelerate discussion in the patient and doctor consultation process by helping physicians focus on diagnostic and therapeutic questions. A tele-medicine consultation process might initiate before the patient physically sits with a care provider such that time is focused on patient concerns and less with preliminaries. While these processes may not be an absolute requirement (not everyone will be comfortable with such a process), it is possible that third-party payors or insurance companies might create financial incentives in exchange for the patient's efforts to actively participate in the healthcare process.

For example, the I3 Consortium (i3.usc.edu) is creating a data architecture where patients could share their healthcare data and identify who has access to the IoT data generated. Consumers who are concerned with community health issues will have the option to contribute certain aspects of their healthcare data to officials at the public health departments or regulatory agencies. Conceivably, participants may want to activate these data feeds during certain seasons and deactivate at other times. Others with security concerns will opt against participation. Independently, citizens will have the option to send the same data to their local physician for preventative purposes. Perhaps, people may opt to release data to insurance companies in exchange for improved benefits. They may also release data to personal service that monitors their health and well-being outside the managed healthcare environment.

In times of healthcare crises, it will be imperative to have the capability for citizens, healthcare professionals, and government agencies to rapidly reconfigure the data driven healthcare infrastructure and systems through initiatives such as I3 (A consortium developing an opensource Internet-of-Things data governance system based on research from USC-Marshall's Institute for Communications Technology Management and USC's Viterbi School of Engineering), which are positioning themselves to fill that need.

With these systems in place, it is possible that in addition to empowering citizens to be more actively involved in the healthcare data ecosystem, some data processing needs may move outside the already overtaxed government/insurance managed healthcare system.

Generally speaking, most technology-driven advancements occur in compartmentalized and independent bubbles; progress achieved in one sector serves as an enabler for progress in another. Properly implemented, technologies like smartphones, EHRs (Electronic Health Records), and even Wi-Fi, have allowed the healthcare industry to improve the communication for patients, efficiencies for administrators, and returns for shareholders.

For example, building an automated inpatient monitoring system for the hospital can improve operating efficiencies while improving patient care. Further progress can be accomplished if data from other administrative domains and consumer devices could be integrated to create a more holistic perspective. Capitalizing on this untapped data to bring incremental value to the healthcare industry is exceedingly difficult when these systems are run by different administrations who have made independent solution purchasing decisions. Further, integration complexity problems can be expected to increase dramatically as the industry continues to shift to data-driven patient management paradigms. Consider a medical device developer who has created a next generation device that gives rise to a plethora of patient monitoring data. Practically speaking, it is almost impossible for an IoT device developer to contemplate all the different ways the data can be utilized by a healthcare professional. If, instead, data collection devices were independent from applications, a single device can drive multiple different diagnostic applications and the issue becomes one of connecting data generators with data consumers. Concepts like VNA (Vendor Neutral Archives) have begun to move the industry in the right direction by allowing medical images to be filed with EMR systems for independent access by various applications; but this concept must be extended to include other IoT devices as well.

Given the lack of an IoT VNA, today's practice considers an IoT application and the associated IoT devices as a complete system. This practice couples IoT devices to specific applications. However, by linking devices to applications, the net effect is to create a series of IoT application silos that are individually managed. Operationally, this is a complex proposition because staff must be dedicated to each silo or staff members need to become operational generalists that provide basic support to a larger number of applications. This same siloed architecture also limits the healthcare professional's ability to leverage data across a broad infrastructure. If certain applications are only aware of a limited number of IoT devices, it may be necessary to duplicate IoT device deployments if a deployed device is incompatible with a new application.

Some IoT application providers have attempted to solve this dilemma by creating application layer APIs which allows their application to link with another, as long as the other application is willing to accept data from a 3rd party. This creates a manageable hierarchy assuming the number of applications remains small. However, such an architecture begins to operationally suffer as the system scales to support a larger number of applications. Moreover, because the connectivity is dependent on the behavior of the applications, each application can become a reliability/performance choke point. Such stop-gap measures can be expected to proliferate until a VNA-type vision is applied to healthcare IoT.

While VNA philosophies can be utilized to reduce the IoT application silos, they will likely not be able to incorporate consumer-targeted medical data into their archives as native data. Consumer IoT devices do not generally live up to medical device quality standards. Comparing a medical halter monitor to data generated by a consumer device will likely lead to confusion unless the healthcare professional knows the source of the data and the validity/reliability of the data sourced from such a device. Additionally, the behavioral dynamics that govern consumer use of a monitor provided by the doctor for temporary use is far different from the behavioral dynamics at play when a consumer purchased IoT device is continually providing data to a third party. Consumers may expect incentives, direct control, and other benefits to accrue from these devices personally procured from outside the healthcare industry. As an additional complication, these independent devices add another dimension to the security conversation given the open nature of these markets.

The creation of an evolved architecture that allows vendor neutral data stores and integration of consumer and medical data into one repository may require additional extensions to current practices. VNA systems can be integrated into medical record management systems at different points in the information flow. However, inclusion of consumer data into medical data flows implies a need for a tool that can serve to route the IoT data into the medical data space and also route it to one or more consumer-friendly applications. Given that the system needs to support data flows between a variety of end-points, the routing mechanism must be security aware so that misbehaving IoT devices (and applications) can be identified and isolated from the network. In addition, the system must support the creation and management of trusted relationships between data end-points with an appreciation for the fact that trust is a dynamic and very personalized expression of acceptability.

The forces that will drive the shift from an application-centric IoT environment to an infrastructure-centric environment are the same as those that drove the evolution of the Internet, with the only tangible uncertainty being the velocity which drives such changes. It can be argued that the lack of an open IoT infrastructure will confine the majority of health care IoT by the IT department's span of control. That is, if an IT department can enforce specific device and application deployment decisions, the need for an open IoT architecture can be reduced. However, such a dictated IoT support plan limits ecosystem partnerships (linkages to independent clinics, surgery centers, ambulances, etc.), and impedes patient-centric participation (unless the hospital provides all needed IoT devices and support).

In an effort to expand the health care paradigm, it becomes important to look at healthcare in the context of the patient. Rather than diagnosing the patient based on information gathered at the doctor's office, the patient should be able to provide the doctor with information about the environment where they reside, work, and transit. Environmental data, including data from consumer quality IoT devices would allow the doctor to make much more informed healthcare decisions. Further, as healthcare-focused artificial intelligence applications become common place, applying data analytics to the wealth of real-time data about individual patients will become common practice.

The reality of this vision is technologically attainable; however, there are many non-technology driven issues that must be faced and conquered before it can be realized. First, all entities must accept the privacy and manageability of such a system—this is not to say that consumers must change but instead means that systems must evolve to accept working within the individual's privacy domain. This is not an easy or straightforward task in that those who generate this data (via their devices) must be comfortable with the fact that they have control over who can see their data and that they can easily extend or rescind data permissions based on their self-interest. In such a data centric word, patients must be treated as health-care partners where they are providing data in exchange for services; this is a give and take relationship like any other partnership. And, like any such partnership, the amount of sharing that occurs is proportional to the level of trust that exists between the parties, and this trust must be developed and maintained over time for the partnership to be successful.

CONCLUSION

In conclusion, data driven medicine is forcing the industry to step past the concept where the healthcare industry is a closed, regulated industry. If certified healthcare professionals are limited and can consider only management by certified infrastructure managers, their ability to make the best possible recommendations will be limited. The concept of a healthcare ecosystem must be expanded to include a broad spectrum of contributors and user groups. This future healthcare ecosystem should encourage data submission from a wide range of sources provided that the provenance of the data is confirmed and documented. Maximizing the use of the data by providers, health systems, and others while protecting the privacy rights of users is a challenge.

While data from IoT-enabled devices and other sources has the potential to improve outcomes, reduce cost of care, and improve the personalization of medical treatment in developed countries, the global impact of this technical trend is even more compelling. In developing nations, as telecom companies expand bandwidth and speed globally, it is possible for international NGO's to begin projecting medical expertise into developing nations.

Future health care digital networks and physical systems must be accessible both digitally and economically while protecting security and accuracy. These communication technology-driven health devices and networks can improve personal and community-wide health and well-being, regardless of diagnosis, disability, health condition, socio-economic, demographic, or other personal privacy concerns. The on-ramp to improving use of IoT systems for healthcare lies in the creation of a big multi-lane, high-speed, digital on-ramp to the medical information superhighway of the future.

REFERENCES

1. Csail, R. G. (2018, June 12). *Artificial intelligence senses people through walls*. Retrieved from http://news.mit.edu/2018/artificial-intelligence-senses-people-through-walls-0612

2. Medicine, N. (2018, June 26). *Northwestern Medicine receives transformative $25 million gift from the Bluhm Family Charitable Foundation*. Retrieved from https://www.prnewswire.com/news-releases/northwestern-medicine-receives-transformative-25-million-gift-from-the-bluhm-family-charitable-foundation-300671938.html

3. *Artificial intelligence-powered Sugar.IQ™ diabetes management app developed by Medtronic and IBM Watson Health Now commercially available.* (n.d.). Retrieved from http://newsroom.ibm.com/announcements?item=122916

4. UWaterlooNews. (n.d.). *AI and radar technologies could help diabetics manage their disease.* Retrieved from https://eurekalert.org/pub_releases/2018-06/uow-aar062718.php

5. Health, J. (2018, September 14). *Geisinger's Steele Institute for Healthcare Innovation selects Jvion's AI to help transform care delivery.* Retrieved from https://jvion.com/news/press/geisinger-s-steele-institute-for-healthcare-innovation-selects-jvion-s-ai-to-help-transform-care-delivery

6. Hung, A. J. (2018, August 01). *Automated performance metrics and machine learning algorithms for robotic surgery.* Retrieved from https://jamanetwork.com/journals/jamasurgery/article-abstract/2685266

7. McCluskey, M. (2018, June 07). *MIT creates world's first 'psychopath' robot.* Retrieved from http://time.com/5304762/psychopath-robot-reactions/

CHAPTER 3

TRANSFORMING HEALTHCARE WITH ARTIFICIAL INTELLIGENCE

Kevin Yamazaki, Benjamin Nguyen,
Nathaniel Bischoff, and Cassandra Gibson

INTRODUCTION

From initial prenatal analysis through palliative care, from congenital defects to chronic disease management, and within every specialty and primary care, Artificial Intelligence (AI) systems have the possibility to shift the paradigm of medicine to more collaborative and proactive care. AI is already being observed in everyday life [1] but has yet to make the full transition to use in medicine [2]. In the current era of medicine, clinicians are expected to sift through an endless stream of data while recalling their personal experiences to make critical, time-sensitive decisions.

In addition, the electronic medical record (EMR), originally intended as a tool to process billing of a patient's medical care, is now used to keep a longitudinal record of all patient interactions. This tool has become more complex and can take a majority of a physician's time during the day. Physician burnout, often due to the EMR, has been well- documented, and has led to widespread dissatisfaction in the profession.

Transforming Healthcare with Big Data and AI, pages 43–59.
Copyright © 2020 by Information Age Publishing
All rights of reproduction in any form reserved.

With all of these problems related to the collection, organization, analysis, and presentation of data, healthcare can greatly benefit from applications of AI. There have been many attempts to use statistical modeling and expert based systems to try and solve many of medicine's biggest questions, but we are far from a one-size-fits-all solution. Because of the explosion of big data, especially in healthcare, advanced machine learning algorithms, and incredible progresses in computing, the last decade has ushered in a new era in AI. Many researchers, startups, and large companies are eager to bring their expertise to the healthcare community. The use of this technology in medical applications in the next quarter century will lead to the most transformative period in medicine's rich history. This review will cover major topics regarding AI in healthcare and medicine.

A HISTORY OF ARTIFICIAL INTELLIGENCE

Centuries before Minsky established the first formal definition of AI in the 1950s, the seeds of AI can be traced back to the logic-based formulas derived by the Greek philosopher Aristotle. However, modern mathematicians Thomas Bayes, George Boole, and Charles Babbage provided the groundwork for current AI techniques. Bayes is best known for developing the framework on probability in the 1760s used in today's AI [3]. Babbage is known for his Analytic Machine, the precursor to the calculator and computer, which he developed throughout the mid to late 1800s, and Boole is known for Boolean Algebra developed in the mid 1800s, the basis behind classification in AI techniques [4][5]. But it wasn't until in the 1940s when Alan Turing, the British mathematician and computer scientist, developed his theory on computation and computing machines that the possibility of AI became a reality [6]. The term "artificial intelligence" was coined by American computer scientist John McCarthy at the 1956 Dartmouth Conference, composed of mathematicians and scientists [7].

Just two years after the landmark Dartmouth Conference in 1958, Frank Rosenblatt's three- layered Perceptron was theorized and documented, which composed of an input layer, transfer function, and output layer within the computer program [8]. This theory became the foundation for the artificial neural network (ANN), and today's deep learning (DL) algorithms [9]. Following these founding, "golden" years in AI, progress became dormant and research funding was cut in the following decades, which was later named the "AI winter" [10].

Beginning in the final decade of the 20th century, AI programmers started a Renaissance by further advancing machine learning and data mining, two key components of AI. At this time, researchers in this field were focused on man versus machine. In intellectual circles, the discussion centered around computers defeating humans in chess, as this was thought of as a test of intellectualism. This era culminated in IBM's Deep Blue defeating the reigning world chess champion Garry Kasparov in 1997 [11].

The history of AI in medicine can be traced back to the 1960s when initial systems focused on diagnosis and therapy. Stanford's Ted Shortliffe developed an innovative program named MYCIN [12]. MYCIN provided the first framework of a rule-based expert system that leveraged "if-then" rules. It was used to recommend antibiotics for various infectious diseases. Although the MYCIN program was never used in a real-time clinical setting, retrospective studies showed that it was superior to human experts in selecting antibiotics. By collecting work in the field from the 1970s, Peter Szolovits wrote the first textbook, *Artificial Intelligence in Medicine,* in 1982 [13].

Up until the 1990s, most work at the intersection of AI and medicine was concentrated in academic centers like Stanford, MIT, and Pittsburgh in the US, with a few focused centers in Europe. In 1987, the European Society for Artificial Intelligence in Medicine initiated a biennial meeting called "Artificial Intelligence in Medicine" [14]. This conference remains an active meeting for sharing research and advancements in the field. In 2005, the first medical AI course was taught by Szolovits at MIT, marking a milestone in the convergence of AI, clinical education and the field of medicine [15]. By this time, many data scientists outside of healthcare were using more advanced methodologies in AI research, but medical researchers were still utilizing traditional statistics.

The digitization of the electronic health record in the early 21st century created a new paradigm in medicine. Data, on the order of petabytes or 1 million gigabytes, is being collected every year in the medical and healthcare domain. This data, on each one of us, is not utilized to improve patient outcomes or prevent adverse events.

MODELS FOR AI INTERACTION DESIGN

We start with a fundamental discussion—the design of AI experiences. AI is, after all, another digital technology—one that must be used by human beings with their own biases, mental models, and ingrained habits. We define 'AI experience' as the interaction between a human being, and a product that uses AI to generate its outputs. As designers, we believe it imperative that any discussion of artificial intelligence includes a discussion of humankind's inevitable interaction with it. While not all AI systems will interact with human beings, those that touch the healthcare system often must, at least in these early days of AI. Human beings generate the inputs, and human beings make decisions based on the outputs—whether they are on a screen or read to them via a voice assistant.

The field of artificial intelligence would describe the design and development of AI as a practice in rationalism [16]. The dominant perspective during the era of high expectations for the near-term creation of human-like AI, the rationalistic approach, strives to model humans as cognitive machines, whose thought processes can be paralleled in digital computers through the use of algorithms and heuristics. This, of course, acts under the assumption that human logic can be "translated" to formal symbolic representation.

The design perspective, on the other hand, focuses on the ecological aspects of designing for human-computer interactions (HCI). This "design" approach is the way designers adapt to the common state of design challenges: Human behavior often doesn't align with known predictive models. Because a digital design exists at the intersection of the technological and the human, design of AI must focus not only on logical patterns, but also on the adaptive nature of world experience. This adaptive process in design occurs through iteration and testing in order to produce the most usable design. Because humans interpret design in related but unique ways, designers utilize testing over predictions and assumption to analyze the efficacy of a design.

Human-Centered Guidelines for Usable AI

Designs are deemed effective or successful when they are *usable*. When it comes to evaluating the usability of artificial intelligence, the interaction points between human and machine must be analyzed for the following, among many other indications of usability: the ability to instill trust, the ability to help users understand limitations and failures, the relative value and effort involved in using the technology, and the ability of the technology to perform without human biases. These criteria should seem familiar to the healthcare professional, as they are not unlike the ways in which patients and providers define positive healthcare experiences. We'll take a closer look at each of these criteria and their relationship to the healthcare experience, which should help us begin to imagine how artificial intelligence can augment the healthcare setting.

Establish Trust

Much like the physician-patient relationship, a level of trust must be established between a user and intelligent technology. Numerous studies and surveys show that trust between patient and provider is established through different techniques depending on the medical and cultural context. Patients often evaluate the trustworthiness of a provider or team of providers by measuring their actions against a set of expectations. Cultural understandings of professionalism and expectations set directly by the physician's interactions contribute to patient expectations [17]. Trust between patient and provider is an ongoing, dynamic process of evaluation and reevaluation, wherein the patient constantly seeks validation of expectations or means for altering those expectations. Although the trust between provider and patient is a human interaction, the patterns and conditions of trust remain throughout interactions between human and computer.

As mentioned before, the logic patterns of artificial intelligence are not entirely analogous to human thought patterns. Therefore, technologies without established logical transparency tend to appear as a "black box" with magical properties to users—only disappointing and confusing them further when unexpected outcomes occur [18]. For artificial intelligence to establish trust, programs should present models that users can understand. Users should be able to predict the outcome of performing an action using intelligent technology by understanding its process.

For example, voice activated AI such as Amazon Alexa or Google Assistant react to plain spoken language and pattern their responses to match the instructions given. Google Assistant does not require users to say things like, "compute x of Earth, where x=distance from the sun," but rather, "Hey Google, how far is Earth from the sun?" If, for some reason, the technology cannot answer a request, the voice makes it clear that they can't help the user with that request, rather than simply not delivering a response. These micro-interactions make it clear to the user what they can and cannot expect of the device, establishing valuable trust between the user and their intelligent technology.

When artificial intelligence takes on a role in healthcare, the trust between user and machine is of the utmost importance. Patients often rely on technology to demystify the complexities of health, whether they are under the guidance of a physician or not. Although resources compiled for physicians are reliable sources, their models and logic are not as accessible to patients. A trustworthy intelligent technology can provide benefits to both the patients who seek trustworthy, accessible information and the physicians who want their patients to be well-informed and empowered.

Help Users Understand and Remedy Failure

In addition to setting and meeting expectations, technology must also remain transparent about errors and limitations. An error in the output of intelligent technology may or may not be due to input error on the part of the user, but the ultimate goal of artificial intelligence and machine learning is to predict and minimize user error. Technology can learn from user error by recognizing what kind of errors users make and directing them to the correct path. Think of all the times that Google has asked you "Did you mean…" after you spelled something incorrectly in the search bar.

Designers are told to always consider the use and misuse of their products, accounting for error and driving users to the correct flow. Artificial intelligence is no different in this respect. If interaction design focuses on the interactions between human and computer, every type of interaction must be considered, even those that are outside the ideal scenario. Usable intelligent technologies continue to alert users to potential errors and utilize the power of continued input from users to identify common error types and "learn" to correct for them. This is an example of machine learning.

Technology that is not prepared to learn from and help users correct for errors cannot serve the healthcare setting effectively. For example, imagine a database that providers could utilize to sort through recommended prescriptions for a particular condition. The software produces a list of recommended drugs and their dosage based on the user's exact input of patient data. You can imagine a scenario in which a provider inputs the patients' age or weight incorrectly when in a hurry or distracted. The system then returns no recommended prescriptions, given that someone who is 60 years old and only 20 pounds should not take any dosage of any of the medications in the database. The user expected to see recommended prescriptions and doses, but the tool performed otherwise. The model did not take into consideration the realities of a busy physician interacting with the system and did not highlight certain types of data entries as likely errors. Without an understanding of or an easy method to pinpoint and fix the input error, the technology cannot improve, and the experience is no longer useful.

Ensure Value Outweighs Effort

The goal of artificial intelligence is to predict user wants and needs and deliver upon those desires automatically, but there are some instances where that process requires more effort from the user than what it's worth. Users constantly weigh the cost and benefit of using a technology or a feature. In some instances, the process of "asking" for things from intelligent technology requires so much user effort, it minimizes the relative value. One example is programming by demonstration tools, which use artificial intelligence to learn and repeat programmed behaviors. In an ideal world, programming by demonstration (PBD) would allow users to create programs without needing to learn any programming languages. Users could simply demonstrate to the computer what tasks the program should accomplish, in a sort of record-and-repeat fashion. For PBD systems, the cost of use includes invoking the system, teaching it the correct procedure, and supervising its progress. Oftentimes, correcting an error requires starting over from the beginning [19]. This cost, in most cases, far outweighs the benefits of automating a task.

Imagine automating your system to read your calendar and set a reminder to take replenishing dietary supplements following scheduled exercise like a hike or a marathon. You might have to train the system using multiple examples that illustrate the intent, hoping that the ai can interpret your intention and turn it into a successful program. Or, you might decide that it would take less time and effort to simply set your reminder manually when you know you'll be exercising heavily. This is the first decision users make every time they interact with a new technology to perform a task.

Some intelligent technologies, on the other hand, balance effort and value so well, that they've integrated so seamlessly into our lives. A key example is the travel time that our navigation systems predict when we select a destination. We've already become accustomed to using digital navigation, because that technology, at some point in its design evolution, became much easier and more beneficial to use than a paper map. It fits into a user's workflow without adjustment on the part of the user while still delivering significant value.

Because technology is becoming part of a healthcare system shifting toward value-based care, the technology itself must be carefully attuned to the value it's providing, and the costs associated with operating the technology. In healthcare, the concept of "value" is one that differs between each stakeholder's perspective and even between individual patients. Overall, both patients and physicians perceive quality of care to be the most important component of value, followed by cost and customer service [20]. When asked about the burden of responsibility for their health, patients weigh themselves and their healthcare providers equally, indicating some ownership of effort for generating positive health outcomes. These insights about patients' desire for value and understanding of the burden of effort should help ground our understanding of the level of effort required and value provided by artificial intelligence in the healthcare setting. Patients are ready to receive value from their healthcare experience in the form of improved quality and lower cost but are perhaps hesitant to interact with technology that requires them to put forth more perceived effort than their healthcare professional.

Avoid Bias

Disparities in treatment of black versus white bodies by healthcare professionals have famously been examined as a manifestation of subconscious human biases [21]. While physicians often carry unintentional biases into the treatment of patients, developers and designers tend to carry subconscious biases into the formulation of artificial intelligence. These biases bear heavy implications when large systems such as government, health, or criminal justice utilize the technology. In 2016, ProPublica exposed racial biases in a software used to predict risk when sentencing criminals [22]. Although question remains regarding whether an algorithm is less biased on average than the judgement of humans, there remains a clear need for these technologies to be evaluated by stakeholders outside of the software development team [23].

Intelligent technologies have the potential to implement decision-making or assessment practices that remove human bias, but only insofar as they can be designed and evaluated to minimize those biases. Artificial logic might not display obviously biased models, but that does not mean that those biases do not exist in use. The success of an intelligent healthcare future is especially dependent on the ability for applications to enact, enforce, and improve the equal of treatment of patients, improving quality of care for all.

ARTIFICIAL INTELLIGENCE: A TECHNICAL REVIEW

To better understand AI, it is important to both define and understand the fundamentals of the methods behind artificial intelligence. AI starts and ends with data, in its many forms. In fact, it can be said that AI is data science, applied; the discipline of data science is ultimately the practice of using data–driven approaches to create AI systems. The bottom line is that data makes AI possible. Like any raw material, it can be 'consumed' in the training of some AI algorithms (those that use supervised learning methods) and is bought and sold by many companies and organizations. Without data, one cannot build AI systems.

Structured versus Unstructured Data

Structured data refers to data that has a defined data model and is highly organized. Structured data is traditionally numerical or tabular data that can be easily ingested into a machine learning algorithm. *Unstructured* data refers to data not in a specific format, with little organization. For a computer program or database, unstructured data is difficult to use. Text, audio, and images are common examples of unstructured data. In the AI community, there has been dramatic improvement in algorithms designed to transform unstructured data to a structured format or ingest unstructured data in a raw format.

Machine Learning

Machine learning (ML) is a subset of AI and perhaps the most commonly known form of AI in the public sphere, as it involves a machine that learns and changes its inner working (algorithms) to achieve a desired outcome. ML is a field of computer science that uses statistical methods to give computer programs the ability to "evolve" their predictions or decisions without the need to be explicitly programmed to do so. In essence, an ML algorithm is written in a way to continually measure its success of predicting the 'correct' answer, and then changes its internal decision-making process appropriately to increase the likelihood of making the right prediction. ML was first coined by Arthur Samuel in 1959 while creating a program to play checkers and is based on data pattern recognition [24]. ML algorithms can be used to solve different types of problems, such as classification (is this an apple or an orange?), regression (which variable can best predict the risk of a myocardial infarction?), clustering (if somebody likes the TV show Game of Thrones, what other shows do they enjoy?), and dimensionality reduction. In order to achieve those outcomes, one must of course create the ML algorithm. There are many ways to create a machine learning algorithm—these fundamental frameworks include logic programming, decision trees, regression analysis, rule-based decision-making, neural networks, and more.

Machine learning algorithms can be broken up into three major categories: supervised, unsupervised, and reinforcement learning. Supervised learning (SL) algorithms use a mathematical model that can be built using a labeled, dependent variable as a mapping function of the independent variables. In essence, an ML algorithm that is trained with supervised learning is given a set of problems and answers to check itself against. Supervised learning can be used to tackle two types of problems: regression (which variable best predicts the risk of a myocardial infarction?) and classification (is this in apple or an orange?). The construction of supervised learning algorithms involves frameworks such as support vector machines, regression, neural networks, deep learning, naive Bayesian classifiers, and hidden Markov models. The discussion of these frameworks in depth is out of the scope of this chapter.

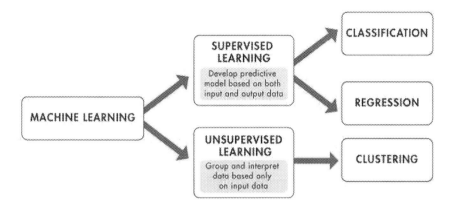

FIGURE 3.1.   Supervised vs. Unsupervised Learning

On the contrary, unsupervised learning (UL) means that there is no dependent variable labeled in the data, and the number of groups (or classes) can varying depending on the data, which can be subject to the discretion of the data scientist. UL can be used to tackle problems such as k-means clustering and principal component analysis [25] [26].

Reinforcement learning (RL) is defined by an agent that makes an action and can change state based on the result of the action in a specific environment. RL is particularly suited for situations where there is a short term, long term trade-off. It includes algorithms such as Monte Carlo models, brute force, and value functions. The use of SL, UL, and RL or a combination of any of the methods is driven by the nature of the question and data of the problem.

Artificial Neural Networks

Artificial neural networks (ANN), or neural networks in the computer science community, are a subset of ML methods wherein the architecture of the algorithm is modeled after the neuronal pathways in the animal brain. This set of methods "learns" by examples without task specific programming by mapping data to labels. An architecture of the ANN is described and then fed using training examples, which the ANN model begins to classify or fit a new example to a certain label—adjusting itself as it receives feedback on its 'correctness.' An ANN's algorithmic structure consists of an input layer, a single hidden layer, and output layer. Like an animal neuron, the hidden layer can take multiple inputs, but generates only one output. An ANN essentially is an algorithm that can take in multiple inputs, each of varying importance, and then make a prediction based on the various inputs, their magnitude, and their relative weights.

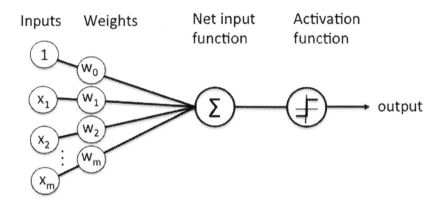

FIGURE 3.2. Artificial Neural Network Structure

Deep Learning

Deep learning (DL) is a subset of ANN in which there is more than one hidden layer in the ANN. Thus, the same general principles apply, except that each hidden layer's output becomes the next hidden layer's input, thus adding significant dimensionality to the predictive power of the algorithm. DL is used in many applications such as image recognition, speech translation and recognition.

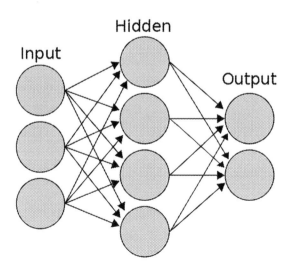

FIGURE 3.3. Deep Learning Structure

Deep learning is presently one of the most commonly utilized methods in AI. There are many different methods being developed and refined every day. In this review, we will cover some of the basic architecture of deep learning. Deep Neural Networks (DNN) are the most general form of DL and consists of more than one hidden layer. Like an actual collection of human neurons, each layer of nodes, characterized by the circles above, trains on a distinct set of features based on the previous layer's output, characterized by the arrows in figure above. Thus, much like the human nervous system, outputs from upstream neurons can be summed to generate a stimulus in downstream neurons. The collective neural network eventually drives towards a decision based on the inputs received from the upstream layers. The most common applications of DNN in healthcare are used in tabular or structured data.

Convolutional Neural Networks (CNN) are as subset of neural networks that leverage convolutions, or the overlap of two functions, to structure the contents of the data. CNN's are most common in image and video analysis and are used extensively in medical imaging processing.

Recurrent Neural Networks (RNN) are a set of networks that use a feedback loop to predict the next step. Because of this unique property, RNN's are common in time- dependent data, audio and text data.

Generative Adversarial Networks (GANs) is a deep neural network architecture that has two networks compete against each other. They are used in the creation of new content (images, text, tabular data) by understanding each individual class.

In the past decade, there have been research and applications in each of these algorithms to continue to improve them and better understand how they work, but it is important to understand the rich history of AI.

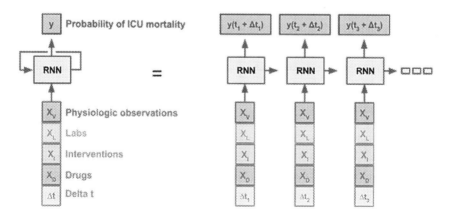

FIGURE 3.4.   Recurrent Neural Network Structure

USE CASES FOR AI IN MEDICINE

In the last five years, multiple factors have led to increased attention and work in AI in general. There have been simultaneous advancements in data storage capacity, computational power and cloud computing along with the development of advanced machine learning algorithms [27]. Cloud data centers and more capable on-premise systems allow for Petabyte (Pb or 1 million Gigabytes) of data to be stored. By using graphics processing unit (GPU) This perfect storm has allowed AI's potential to be more deeply realized. Many large companies including Google, IBM, Apple and Microsoft, and research institutions like Stanford, MIT and UCSF, have partnered with healthcare institutions or created their own divisions dedicated to advancing AI in medicine. Decades old problems in medicine that remain unanswered due to their complex, unique, and heterogeneous nature can now be addressed.

Recently, AI systems have been developed to solve some of humanity's toughest challenges. Most recently, in 2016, Google's DeepMind AlphaGo program defeated the human Go champion Lee Sedol, proving that the computer leveraging deep learning can reach new heights and further advance AI. In 2017, AlphaGo Zero, an updated product by DeepMind, mastered superhuman proficiency in Go without human input [28].

The transition from human cognitive games and puzzles has not translated well to the healthcare domain, however. Currently, clinical and non-clinical healthcare data resides in many silos and is not conducive to using these AI tools. In healthcare, emerging data sources are less structured and inconsistent [29]. In addition, real-time data analysis can be difficult because AI learns from existing questions and data. Many healthcare organizations, and Electronic Health Record (EHR) vendors are focused on organizing and consolidating data for future use of machine learning. In the past decade, Health Level Seven International (HL-7) and Fast Healthcare Interoperability Resources (FHIR) have become standard for data storing and transfer in the healthcare community. As data in healthcare becomes more centralized and industry leaders have begun to focus their sights on AI in healthcare, it is important to see how the medical community can interact with AI systems and software.

AI in Critical Care

One area of growing interest for artificial intelligence in medicine is in the domain of critical care. There are a number of different factors that have led to the increased focus in this area including diversity and volume of data, clinical problems in need of new solutions, and collaborations between institutions.

Machine learning solutions are only as good as the data that is collected and curated. Due to the severity and fluctuation of the condition of patients in the intensive care units (ICUs), ICUs collect a wide variety of data at a higher rate as compared to general medical units. ICU settings are a great opportunity for data scientists to solve clinical problems using machine learning. Some types of data such as vital sign data (heart rate, respiratory rate, and blood pressure) are continuously collected and stored for training machine learning models. Because patients are constantly monitored, hospital data scientists and clinical staff can deploy the models. The diversity of data can include medications, laboratory results, documentation, and other types of data. This data, when brought together intelligently, provides an opportunity to gain powerful insights to predict adverse events and situations where patients can be moved to another medical unit of the hospital or discharged from the hospital. Etiometry, a startup in Massachusetts, has developed an FDA- approved platform to ingest all of this data and present the machine-learned results in an intuitive way.

There is currently a need for new solutions in the intensive care units due to the complexity of these patients and the time sensitive nature of their condition. Clinical decision support (CDS) tools and severity scores have been employed in many hospital settings, but often these systems are limited in their nature to evolve over time, both a factor of their initial scope and regulatory restrictions. There are now a number of learning algorithms that have been developed and are currently being validated for clinical use in the critical care setting. Algorithms developed for the prediction of sepsis, adverse cardiac and respiratory events, and severity score are in the validation stages at several institutions around the United States. These algorithms have been trained in- house at hospital institutions and third-party companies around the world.

Finally, there have been some collaborative efforts to push the boundaries in critical care AI. Medical Information Mart for Intensive Care (MIMIC) "is an openly available dataset developed by the MIT Lab for Computational Physiology, comprising de-identified health data associated with ~40,000 critical care patients. It includes demographics, vital signs, laboratory tests, medications, and more." The team at the MIT Lab has been traveling around the world hosting "datathons" to create new insights and an interface for data scientists and clinicians to work together. The Virtual Pediatric Intensive Care Unit (VPICU) at Children's Hospital of Los Angeles created the PICU Data Collaborative. The PICU Data Collaborative collects critical care EMR data from member hospitals, and the members can decide which problems they will solve and collaborate on algorithm development.

In order to fully realize the potential of AI within the critical care domain of medicine, collaboration among medical institutions, academia and industry must continue to grow. Organizations must test algorithms claiming to beat the gold standard by clinical validation.

AI in Medical Imaging

Artificial intelligence has ushered a new age in medical imaging. In recent years, many different types of organizations have been involved in the advancement of medical imaging through AI. Large medical companies like Siemens have focused on machine learning in image acquisition to direct their machines to take better images at optimal angles. Large tech companies such as NVIDIA have been advocating for medical image analysis using their graphics processing cards. Google has released a number of studies looking at predicting retinopathy using imaging-based machine learning. Startups like Arterys have developed solutions to analyze cardiac, lung, and liver images for segmentation and diagnosis. Academic centers and hospital organizations such as the Center for Clinical Data Science at Mass General and Brigham and Women's Hospital are working on cutting edge solutions for image analysis in a number of different areas. The University of California at Irvine launched the Center for Artificial Intelligence in Diagnostic Medicine to focus on applying machine learning for patient care. The Center was started by two clinicians who had trained in neuroradiology and were applying technology they had developed to analyze head CT scans.

The NIH and FDA has sponsored challenges for individuals and organizations by releasing open datasets to the public to find innovate solutions. These vast datasets have allowed academic labs and individuals to get involved and apply their knowledge base to the domain of medical imaging. This introduced the concept of transfer learning, machine learning in which you learn characteristics such as edges, lines, and features from another domain of images. This strategy has led to positive results in some cases. It has also sparked dialogue between clinicians and data scientists about the role of AI in medical care. Many prominent data scientists have been quoted saying that machine learning algorithms will replace the need for radiologists to interpret images. Radiologists have fallen into two camps in recent years, those who are willing to adopt and advocate for this technology and those who reject the idea that this technology can be beneficial to their work. Professional societies in radiology such as the Radiological Society of North America have begun to highlight and facilitate those working on AI in medical imaging in their publications and meetings.

Medical imaging machine learning techniques employ convolutional neural networks (CNNs). CNNs apply filters to look for lines, edges, shapes, and spatial differences to look for patterns in the images. These patterns are then correlated to different classes (i.e. the presence or absence of an aneurysm in a head CT scan).

Medical imaging has quickly become the most popular use case for AI in healthcare, as the field of imaging, by virtue of the technological infrastructure employed, tends to have all the required components readily available for the development of modern AI systems. These systems have a wealth of labeled data, GPU cards for image processing, and pioneers are beginning to explore the utilization of deep and transfer learning networks.

AI in Medical Administrative Tasks

Issues around the effects of medical administrative tasks have been well documented in recent years. The burden of maintaining correct and thorough documentation takes up a majority of health care professionals' time. Determining the correct course of necessary care has become increasingly difficult due to complexity in medical record organization and procedural processes. Keeping up with current medical literature to make sure standards are up to date has become almost impossible. All these concepts in principle, such as increased information on each patient and knowledge discovery in the research community, should lead to more personalized and correct decision making. However, there has been a failure of the medical community to organize and present the information in a coherent way that does not affect the workflow of members in the care team. This effect paired with increased pressure on physicians and nurses to see more patients in less time, has led to burnout and mental health issues within members of the medical community and poorer care of patients.

Because of the volume of awareness in the medical community, solutions have been proposed using machine learning and artificial intelligence to address issues at the root of the problem. Companies such as Olive are working on mapping the healthcare journey in order to fix problems such as prior authorizations with insurance and billing for care. This combines "classic" machine learning such as expert systems that can make decisions on repeatable tasks, with "new" artificial intelligence by using neural networks to predict new decisions. Augmedix, a startup in San Francisco, California, is working on automated documentation using augmented reality from Google Glass. This solution uses multiple forms of AI such as voice recognition, natural language processing, and feature mapping to present the information back to the clinician in real time. This underscores a pattern of technology companies taking on the challenge of leveraging natural language processing and automatic speech recognition to streamline the clinical documentation workflow. Insurance companies like Alignment Healthcare and Oscar Healthcare are using machine learning to personalize health plans, and track patients during their journey to ensure they are getting the best care.

For the data science community, the role of the medical community (physicians, nurses, patients, family members, and other patient care providers) is to provide input for the problems that are most pressing in the medical community, truth behind the data being analyzed, and guidance when looking at results.

REFERENCES

1. Appenzeller, T. (2017). How AI is transforming science. *Science, 357*(6346), 16–17.
2. Shapshay, S. M. (2014). Artificial intelligence: The future of medicine? *JAMA Otolaryngol Head Neck Surg, 140*(3), 191.
3. Bayes, T., Price, R., & Canton, J. (1763). *An essay towards solving a problem in the doctrine of chances.* Royal Society of Publishing
4. Boole, G. (1847). *The mathematical analysis of logic.* Cambridge, MA: Cambridge University Press.
5. Boole, G. (1854). *An investigation of the laws of thought on which are founded the mathematical theories of logic and probabilities.* New York, NY: Macmillan.
6. Copeland, B. R., & Taylor M. S. (2004). Trade, growth, and the environment. *Journal of Economic Literature, 42*(1), 7–71.

7. McCarthy, J., Minsky, M. L., Rochester, N., & Shannon, C. E. (1955). A proposal for the Dartmouth summer research project on artificial intelligence. *AI Magazine, 27*(4), 12–14.

8. Rosenblatt, F. (1958). The perceptron: A probabilistic model for information storage and organization in the brain. *Psychological Review, 65*(6), 386–408.

9. LeCun, Y., Bengio, Y., & Hinton, G. (2015). Deep learning. *Nature, 521*(7553), 436–44.

10. National Research Council. (1966). *Language and machines: Computers in translation and linguistics*. Washington, DC: The National Academies Press. https://doi.org/10.17226/9547

11. Kasparov, G., & Greengard, M. (1996). *Deep thinking: Where machine intelligence ends and human creativity begins*. New York, NY: PublicAffairs.

12. Shortliffe, E. (1975). A model of inexact reasoning in medicine. *Mathematical Biosciences, 23*(3–4), 351–379.

13. Szolovits, P. (1982). Artificial intelligence methods for medical expert systems. *Proc. Amer. Med. Informatics Assn. Congress 82*.

14. Posenato, R. (2019). Home. *Artificial intelligence in medicine (AIME)*. Retrieved from: http://aime17.aimedicine.info/images/PDF/AIME17-Program.pdf

15. Ohno-Machado, L. (2005). *HST.947 medical artificial intelligence*. Boston, MA: MIT OpenCourseWare.

16. Winograd, T. (2006). Shifting viewpoints: Artificial intelligence and human–computer interaction. *Artificial Intelligence, 170*(18), 1256–1258. doi:10.1016/j.artint.2006.10.011

17. Hupcey, J., Penrod, J., & Morse, J. (2000). Establishing and maintaining trust during acute care hospitalizations. *Scholarly Inquiry for Nursing Practice, 14*, 227–42.

18. Dove, G., & Halskov, K. (2017). UX design innovation: Challenges for working with machine learning as a design material. *Proceedings of the 2017 CHI Conference on Human Factors in Computing Systems—CHI 17*. doi:10.1145/3025453.3025739

19. Nie, Y., & Lau, S. (2009). Complementary roles of care and behavioral control in classroom management: The self-determination theory perspective. *Contemporary Educational Psychology, 34*, 185–194.

20. Bringing value into focus: The state of value in U.S. healthcare [Scholarly project]. (2017, November). In *Utah health: The state of value in U.S. healthcare*. Retrieved September 11, 2018, from https://uofuhealth.utah.edu/value

21. Hoffman, K. M., Trawalter, S., Axt, J. R., & Oliver, M. N. (2016). Racial bias in pain assessment and treatment recommendations, and false beliefs about biological differences between blacks and whites. *Proceedings of the National Academy of Sciences of the United States of America, 113*(16), 4296–4301. Retrieved from: http://doi.org/10.1073/pnas.1516047113

22. Angwin, J. (2016). *Machine bias: There's software used across the country to predict future criminals. And it's biased against blacks*. Retrieved from: https://www.propublica.org/article/machine-bias-risk-assessments-in-criminal-sentencing

23. Spielkamp, M. (June, 2017). We need to shine more light on algorithms so they can help reduce bias, not perpetuate it. *MIT Technology Review, 16*. Retrieved from: www.technologyrev iew.com/s/607955/inspecting-algorithms-for-bias/

24. Samuel, A. L. (1959). Some studies in machine learning using the game of checkers. *IBM Journal of Research and Development, 44*, 206–226.

25. Hutson, M. (2017). AI glossary: Artificial intelligence, in so many words. *Science, 357*(6346), 19.
26. Hutson, M. (2017). AI in action: How algorithms can analyze the mood of the masses. *Science, 357*(6346), 23–23.
27. Griebel, L. et al. (19 Mar. 2015). A scoping review of cloud computing in healthcare. *BMC medical informatics and decision making.* BioMed Central. Retrieved from: www.ncbi.nlm.nih.gov/pubmed/25888747
28. Silver D., Huang, A., & Maddison, C. J. (2016). Mastering the game of Go with deep neural networks and tree search. *Nature, 529*, 484–489.
29. Chen J. H., & Asch, S. M. (2017). Machine learning and prediction in medicine — Beyond the peak of inflated expectations. *New Engl. J. Med., 376*(26), 2507–2509.

CHAPTER 4

THE APPLICATIONS OF BLOCKCHAIN IN HEALTHCARE

Hugh Gordon

Blockchain, the technology behind cryptocurrencies like Bitcoin and Ethereum, has enormous potential that is just beginning to be explored. The concept of a secure distributed ledger—a source of truth that can't be altered by any one entity—is compelling to say the least. Outside of cryptocurrencies, healthcare is another field where blockchain could make remarkable improvements. The combination of tremendously valuable, highly private information, a high degree of regulation and many interested parties found in healthcare today creates a perfect storm of bureaucracy and red tape. Blockchain has the potential to significantly alter healthcare methodologies by radically increasing transparency, leading to greater efficiency and more trust in the healthcare system.

In this chapter, we will explain the history and technical basics of blockchain, developing a working knowledge of the concepts and technology behind blockchain. On this foundation, we will build an understanding of the current state of blockchain in healthcare using a series of practical, example-based explanations. Finally, we will discuss challenges and future possibilities for blockchain in healthcare.

Transforming Healthcare with Big Data and AI, pages 61–75.

THE NEED FOR BLOCKCHAIN IN HEALTHCARE

Healthcare is a unique industry in many ways, and this is reflected in the complexities of interacting with healthcare data. The industry's sheer scale, heavy regulation, and security requirements make healthcare data complicated and often inefficient. Technologies like blockchain have the potential to simplify some of these processes, making working with healthcare data easier and more efficient. The largest areas of impact are maintaining the security of health data and simplifying the bewildering array of regulations and data standards that exist in healthcare today.

Security

One of healthcare data's greatest difficulties is the required high degree of security. The cost of a data breach is high both in terms of financial liability and in the effect that a breach could potentially have on individual lives. Medical records often contain information that can be devastating to patients if shared improperly, such as HIV status or medication details. Additionally, health records contain billing information which is critical to both providers and payers. The combination of sensitivity to patients and the value of the data makes security a top priority. While blockchain was built with the banking and monetary systems in mind, the underlying principles of information security extend across industries and, in turn, so can its usefulness in providing security.

Information security is defined in United States law as: "the protection of information and systems from unauthorized access, use, disclosure, disruption, modification, or destruction in order to provide confidentiality, integrity, and availability." [1] The key pieces of this definition are the provision of confidentiality, integrity, and availability. Known by its initials inside the information security community as the CIA triad, these three features are an essential part of any information security regimen. They define what it is for something to be "secure." In healthcare, these three features are critical and blockchain offers solutions to help improve each one.

Confidentiality

Confidentiality is perhaps the easiest information security principal to apply to healthcare. Simply put, healthcare data is private, and it is crucial that only appropriately authorized individuals have access to it. This was enshrined into US law with the Health Insurance Portability and Accountability Act of 1996 (HIPAA). While in principle this sounds fairly straightforward, in practice it is nontrivial: the US government estimates the total cost of HIPAA to be $114 million–225.4 million per year [2].

A great example of the importance of confidentiality in dealing with health records is HIV or any other chronic illness status. Patient's trust providers and insurance companies to keep this information private and releasing this information to the wrong party can have tremendous consequences for both patients and providers alike.

Integrity

Healthcare systems operate in an environment where trust between various parties can be difficult and hard to achieve. Insurance companies must trust that healthcare providers are billing correctly; patients must believe that they are getting appropriate care. Nobody wants fraudulent medical records or billing practices to occur, and that starts with strong assurances of data integrity. Having strong assurance of data integrity is a cornerstone of trust, and to that end, today, every transaction or agreement in healthcare is hampered by time-intensive and expensive processes that are necessary to ensure security [3].

For instance, providers don't trust insurers to reimburse for procedures, and increasingly, even to cover them in the first place. Due to changing regulations and healthcare markets in the U.S., many healthcare providers frequently change the insurance they accept and the terms they accept it under. Additionally, insurance companies don't trust providers, regularly contesting claims and adding to providers' administrative burdens. The American Medical Association estimates that inefficient claims processing costs 10–14% of practice revenue [4]. Patient trust in healthcare providers is also highly variable, depending on demographic factors as well as the clinical situation. Finally, patient trust in health insurance is abysmal: yearly results of the Harris Poll have consistently shown it's one of the least trusted industries, placing alongside tobacco and coal in consumer trust [5, 6].

To illustrate how much friction ensuring data integrity can add to the healthcare system, consider the example of physician credentialing. It can take months for a physician moving to a new state to transfer credentials, and this is solely due to the time and effort spent ensuring the integrity of the physician's credentials. Let's say a doctor wants to work at a hospital in another state where doctors are more needed, so she applies and gets accepted. Could she start working there next month? No, because credentialing the doctor according to regulations in the new state takes an average of six months. These regulations are put in place to protect patients—you wouldn't want your doctor to be practicing medicine without board certification. However, for doctors, this makes career moves more difficult than most other professionals, and it contributes to the global shortage of doctors. The Association of American Medical Colleges reports that by 2025, the United States alone will be short 90,400 doctors [7].

Prior authorization—ensuring the integrity of a request for a procedure or treatment before paying for it is another example of friction added to the system.

Availability

The availability of healthcare data is essential but often overlooked. The medical record is not only important to understand the clinical status of a patient, but also for research purposes and as a legal document that protects both patients and providers. In order for it to be at all useful, however, the information needs to be available. HIPAA mandates six years of availability—that is all protected health information must be kept (or available) for six years after its creation and provided upon request to patients, auditors or other healthcare providers.

For example, data availability in an emergency can mean the difference between life and death. In the case of a flu epidemic, for instance, it's imperative that data regarding the spread and treatment of the current strain is made available to the FDA and other governing bodies so that they can help allocate crucial public health resources. Just as importantly, data regarding the appropriate treatment of a novel disease or strain must be made available to providers so that they can treat appropriately. This availability problem rose to enough prominence during a recent flu epidemic that the FDA is now designing a blockchain based system, RAPID, to ensure fast data sharing in an emergency.

To sum it all up, the distributed ledger with well-defined state transitions provided by blockchain is an ideal technology to remove some of the friction added to healthcare by the high-security requirements. It provides a foundational toolset of concepts that can be used to ensure the security of and reduce the friction of working with sensitive health data.

Regulation and Fragmentation

To varying degrees in healthcare systems around the world, legal and regulatory barriers initially intended to protect patients are now preventing devastatingly needed innovation in care delivery.

Fragmented approaches to healthcare management have been an expensive and growing problem for decades. In 2010, the World Health Organization published a global study of health systems financing, which found that "conservatively speaking, about 20–40% of resources spent on health are wasted, resources that could be redirected towards achieving universal coverage" [8]. They find the main culprit to be medicines—expensive brands over generics, antibiotic and injection overuse, poor storage, and wide variations in price—but this waste also includes inefficient hospital processes, medical errors, underutilized or inefficiently used technologies, and the way service providers are paid. Fee-for-service payment structures tend to over-serve those who can pay and under-serve those who cannot. In addition, local laws and regulations reduce the availability of health data generated or recorded in each location, but even if it was available data, it would be so complicated and fragmented that no one can even use it.

Health Data is Fragmented, Inaccessible, and Incomplete

Data is the foundation for insights and the development of healthcare innovations. Yet, when compared to other industries, healthcare has been slow to benefit due to the entrenched problem of incomplete and inaccessible data across organizations. Until recently, healthcare records have been primarily stored on paper; electronic health records (EHRs) are relatively new. There are many problems with EHRs, but chief among them is data quality and the fact that these EHRs are housed within healthcare systems where hospitals, not patients, are in control of the data. However, healthcare consumers are mobile. They may visit multiple doctors in various institutions by choice or by forced circumstance, and their data does not travel with them. In fact, regulation around data privacy, intended to protect patients, has led to both significant healthcare waste and patient harm in the form of treatment delays and errors, as well as over-testing and inappropriate testing. It is important to note that the structure and focus of EHRs are not on accurate and effective recording of data for the patient and their wellbeing, but on medical billing. This situation has led to patient data being spread out across multiple silos; inaccessible to both patients and their providers.

It is indisputable that EHRs have improved medical communication, but this process remains far from ideal [9]. There exist few incentives and many disincentives for parties in healthcare to share data, and patients who need their data exchanged quickly between providers are often left waiting or forced to repeat expensive and sometimes invasive tests. In the worst case, healthcare suffers because providers have an incomplete picture of patients' health status. Exchanging data between providers can take weeks and significant effort on behalf of the provider and patient. Records are often sent via mail or fax (which in any other industry would be considered antiquated) which merely aggravates the problem.

Furthermore, as mentioned above, EHRs are woefully incomplete. Providers do not have the time or incentive to enter accurate or complete data, and data is only recorded when healthcare consumers are physically present. Increasingly abundant health data collected via digital health products and services in between physician visits is rarely incorporated into a person's treatment plan, and the full incorporation of such data would likely require an architectural overhaul of most EHRs. EHRs are just not designed to manage multi-institutional, lifetime medical records. Patients leave data scattered across various organizations, and there is no system in place to connect the dots from a data perspective. This prevents patients from having easy access to past data, as the provider, not the patient, generally retains primary stewardship (either through explicit legal means in over 21 states or simply because it's too much hassle for the patient to retrieve their record) [10]. This leaves data fragmented and incomplete with neither providers nor patients having a complete picture of the patient's health.

Additionally, the HIPAA privacy rule allows providers to take up to 60 days to respond to a patient's request to change inaccurate data. [11]. Beyond this time delay and the difficulty in correcting one's record, record maintenance can prove challenging to initiate as patients are not encouraged or enabled to review their full record [10, 11]. Patients thus interact with records in a fractured manner that reflects the nature of EHR management.

The Challenge of Data Sharing

Interoperability challenges between different provider and hospital systems pose additional barriers to effective data sharing. This lack of coordinated data management and exchange means health records are fragmented, rather than cohesive [12]. Patients and providers may face significant hurdles in initiating data retrieval and sharing due to providers' economic incentives that encourage "health information blocking." The office of the national coordinator (ONC) is responsible for coordinating and regulating EHRs in the United States. An ONC report details several examples on this topic, namely health IT developers interfering with the flow of data by charging exorbitant prices for data exchange interfaces [13]. When designing new systems to overcome these barriers, we must prioritize patient agency. Patients benefit from a holistic, transparent picture of their medical history [12]. This is crucial in establishing trust and continued participation in the medical system, as patients that doubt the confidentiality of their records may abstain from full, honest disclosures or even avoid treatment. In the age of online banking and social media, patients are increasingly willing, able and desirous of managing their data on the web and on the go [12]. However, proposed systems must also recognize that not all provider records can or should be made available to patients (i.e., provider psychotherapy notes, or physician intellectual property), and should remain flexible regarding such record-onboarding exceptions [14, 15]. There also is few provision in current systems for research and public health which rely on healthcare data to make forward progress.

Medical records are critical for research and public health. The ONC's report emphasizes that biomedical and public health researchers "require the ability to analyze information from many sources in order to identify public health risks, develop new treatments and cures, and enable precision medicine" [13]. Though some data trickles through to researchers from clinical studies, surveys and teaching hospitals, we note a growing interest among patients, care providers and regulatory bodies to responsibly share more data, and thus enable better care for others [13, 16]

Both maintaining appropriate security and working within the patchwork of regulations are critical pieces of working with health data that need serious improvement. Blockchain-based technologies are being deployed to help cope with these security and data quality issues.

BLOCKCHAIN FUNDAMENTALS

Popularized by Bitcoin, blockchain is a description of a group of computational protocols that allow for the creation and maintenance of a distributed ledger with built-in features to avoid tampering by any one individual. Technically speaking, blockchains rely on computational proof of work to achieve consensus, which means that the majority of participants in a given block chain have to agree that a given transaction is valid before it can be added to the ledger. While blockchain was initially created to serve as the technological framework for Bitcoin, a digital currency, it has since spread with applications in everything from manufacturing to government and healthcare.

History

The concept of decentralizing currency was formally proposed in 1974 by F. A. Hayek as a method to stop inflation and provide for a low friction means of international trade [17]. The 1980s and 1990s saw the development of e-cash protocols that provided anonymity but still relied on a centralized party. In 1998 b-money was proposed by Wei Bai as a framework of how to create a distributed currency using computational puzzles to achieve consensus [18]. It wasn't until 2009 that Satoshi Nakamoto took all these ideas and created Bitcoin, a purely peer-to-peer (meaning no middlemen involved, unlike banking transactions or systems like PayPal) version of electronic cash [19]. The breakthrough that Satoshi made was the creation of a consensus algorithm that used cryptographic primitives, the building blocks of cryptography and most secure systems, to allow participants in the peer-to-peer network to demonstrate proof of work and then come to a consensus without any centralized authority. The lack of centralized authority is critical to blockchain as it allows participation in the network to be open to anyone, without a formal barrier to entry (such as registration) but still keep the consensus from undue influence or technical attacks [20]. Bitcoin is centered solely around the idea of currency and currency exchange, and other alternative ideas for using the underlying blockchain technology existed creating more complicated financial instruments and allowing for a permissioned or private blockchain. Technologies like Ethereum and HyperLedger arose to fill those needs.

Technical Underpinnings

A blockchain is an append-only distributed ledger that shares data among participants. The only way to update or add a transaction to the ledger is to provide proof of work or proof of stake, which proves that a majority of the blockchain participants believe that the transaction is valid.

Generalized Blockchain Architecture

The blockchain is a sequence of blocks each of which holds a list of transactions. These blocks are linked together into a chain as each block has the cryptographic hash of the previous one stored in its header. Each user of the blockchain has a public key and private key. After a new transaction is created, the user signs the transaction with their private key, and then the transaction is verified by a peer user. The transaction is certified by using the user's public key to verify that the signature is valid. Once an appropriate number of users have verified the transaction, it becomes part of the current block. This process is then repeated for each transaction. This results in a chain of transactions, broken up into blocks, with the following properties: decentralization, persistence, anonymity, and auditabil-

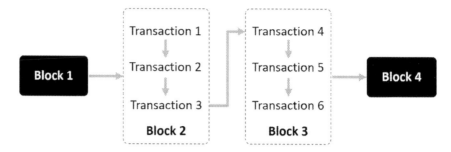

FIGURE 4.1. Generic Blockchain: Transactions are Grouped in Blocks and Linked Together to Form a Chain

ity [21]. These properties are the things that set blockchain apart from a simple ledger, so here we'll discuss them in detail.

- **Decentralization:** In a typical transaction system, such as real property title or transactions in a bank account, each transaction needs to be verified by a centralized authority such as a bank or government before being placed in the ledger. As long as the centralized party is trusted, this assures that the transaction is valid. However, it also provides a single point of vfailure, and there is no fail-safe if the trusted centralized party records an incorrect transaction. In a blockchain, every party to the chain may verify any transaction, and a transaction only becomes official after a consensus is reached that the transaction is correct. This way, no one entity can modify the chain.
- **Persistency:** In a traditional ledger, there is usually a single master copy. For instance, in the case of real property, the title is stored at a government office. In a blockchain, each user can maintain a full copy of all transactions. This eliminates the concept of an 'original' and eliminates the risk of losing the data associated with the blockchain.
- **Anonymity:** Blockchain users are identified solely by their public keys (which can be thought of like a very long ID number). This means that there is no concept of identity, aside from a long random number, associated with each transaction. Additionally, it is only possible to prove that a given user is authorized to make transactions on a given public key if they have the private key. This creates a situation where there is no way to definitively link the real identity of a given user with a real person or entity. A corollary of this that is relevant to healthcare is that there is also no recourse for a user who loses their key built into the blockchain system.
- **Auditability:** The blockchain can be thought of as a state machine: each transaction is a well-defined transition from a previous state to a new state. Each transaction is also associated, indelibly, with a given public key and

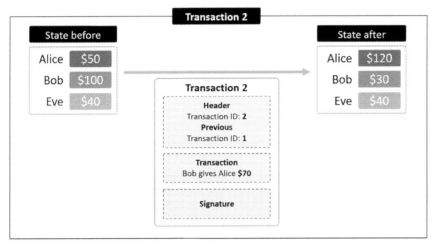

FIGURE 4.2   Example Transaction: Bob Gives Alice $70

a timestamp. This means that it's possible to trace precisely how each user came to possess the balance that they now have, and it's impossible to have unexplained or illegal transactions. This is very relevant for healthcare as it is possible to prove which user(s) authorized which transaction mathematically. For instance, in the case of a prescription for a controlled substance, it would be possible to prove which health care provider authorized it, substantially reducing (almost eliminating) the possibility of fraud.

Special Characteristics

Not all blockchains are the same. The original, Bitcoin, is simply a ledger containing records of the exchange of digital currency. There are many variations on that original theme but two, smart contracts and permissioned blockchains, are particularly relevant to healthcare.

- **Smart Contracts:** Bitcoin was built with a basic set of operations: each transaction contains a set of inputs (defined as a number of coins and an associated account) and a set of outputs. This allows for the exchange of money with transactions like "User A gives 5 coins to user B," but that is the extent of the functionality. There are many more transactions, or contracts, one may wish to write. For instance, "User A gives 50% of his house to user B if user B gives 20 coins to user A in the next two days." Other implementations of the blockchain attempt to provide this functionality. The most well-known one, Ethereum, attempts to build a generalized, secure, transaction-based state machine [22]. This leads to a de facto secure, distributed computation framework which is very useful in the context of healthcare.

- **Permissioned Blockchains:** Another feature that Bitcoin lacks is the idea of permissions. Bitcoin works like any real-world currency: if you possess coins, you can hold them, spend them, or give them to anyone else without any rules. However, when considering the usage of blockchain outside of simple currency transactions, like in healthcare, the idea of rules or permissions becomes essential. The ability to dictate who can see the blockchain and who may perform transactions is very desirable. Hyperledger Fabric is perhaps the most well-known permissioned blockchain technology, allowing for non-sequential execution of transactions and the execution of specific transactions on specific sets of machines. This allows for confidentiality while maintaining the previously stated advantages of blockchain [23].

BLOCKCHAIN APPLICATIONS IN HEALTHCARE

Blockchain has broad applicability in healthcare to help tackle the problems of providing adequate security and adherence to regulations while allowing for a rapid pace of innovation and less per transaction cost. There are four major categories of project types out there currently.

Monetizing Personal Health Data

The ability to control the flow of and benefit from the monetization of your personal health data is a concept that is foreign to most people but, if you think about it, it should be commonplace. Currently, health data is monetized mostly without thought to the patient, as the transaction cost would be prohibitively high. BitMED is an example of a company using blockchain to allow for control and monetization of health data.

The BitMED Health protocol is an open-source, distributed consensus ledger with a native currency, the BXM token. It is designed to prevent double spending in the healthcare system, incentivizes health participation among patients and supports smart contracts, decentralized applications and provides protection for personally identifiable information [24]. The BitMED Health Protocol essentially provides a currency-like representation of healthcare information and the tools to use it. The aim is to incentivize patients to provide their information for use in applications and to provide applications a way to pay for the privilege to use that information. It's a protocol and marketplace for health data.

BitMED allows one to exchange their health data for BXM tokens and then allows one to exchange these tokens for services. The BitMED ecosystem incentivizes the transaction of data between stakeholders. For example, patient data is aggregated, de-identified, and accessed based on conditions set by each contributor. This data may be used for patient care, research, clinical trials, etc. When the data is accessed, the patient that contributed the data gets tokens as defined by a smart contract. The patient then may turn around and use these tokens to receive telehealth services [24].

It's easy to see the benefits provided by such an ecosystem; benefits that only blockchain can fully realize. Patients remain in full control of their data—the exchange of data for tokens is clear—and this transparency and direct incentivization encourages data sharing by patients. By automating much of the compliance and reducing time-consuming manual tasks, transaction costs are lowered allowing data and tokens to flow more freely. This gives researchers, health care providers and others who would use data easy access to accurate health data, the price of which is set by the market. It gives patients a way to derive direct benefit from sharing their data through increased access to services.

This sort of exchange happens today, but it is inefficient and opaque to consumers creating high barriers to entry for would-be users of health data and making the benefits of sharing not at all apparent to patients. The distributed, transparent nature of blockchain allows for ecosystems such as BitMED to exist and flourish.

Healthcare Administration

Demand for healthcare continues to rise throughout the world. A large part of this is the rising cost of providing care. A New England Journal study estimated that 31 percent of healthcare costs in the US could be attributed to administration [25]. A majority of that cost goes towards billing: another study estimated that for every 10 physicians providing care, there are 7 additional people employed providing billing and administration services [26]. The costs of providing healthcare globally continue to outstrip inflation year over year [27]. These inefficiencies and rising costs are creating significant pressure on governments to find ways to provide care more cost-effectively.

Estonia has taken an innovative path to address the rising cost of healthcare: blockchain. In 2016, Estonia saw that blockchain had the potential to increase efficiencies in the provision of healthcare nationally and now, through the Estonian company Guardtime, has used blockchain to secure the health data of its residents [28]. The distributed nature of blockchain has allowed Estonia to ease the sharing of health data among authorized parties within the government. This has increased the coordination of care across various government entities, decreased the costs of billing and simplified auditing health data use [29].

The prototype electronic health record management system, MedRec, found a similar solution to that of Estonia, using blockchain to speed access to medical data, increase interoperability, increase patient agency and improve data quality. Built by researchers at MIT Media Lab and Beth Israel Deaconess Medical Center, Med Rec is a novel, decentralized record management system developed to manage electronic health records (EHRs) using blockchain technology [30]. Using Ethereum smart contracts, MedRec demonstrates how decentralization could feasibly create secure, interoperable EHR systems using a system of open APIs. While more of a concept system, it shows the power of blockchain to break down the data silos that cause so much inefficiency with healthcare administration today.

Prototypes like MedRec or real-world examples like Estonia's nationwide blockchain based medical record all show how providing appropriate security, transparency and patient control of their own health data can break down silos and significantly increase the efficiency of providing healthcare.

Public Health and Research

Another area that is seeing benefit of blockchain technology in healthcare is public health. A great example of this is the Food and Drug Administration's (FDA) RAPID protocol. Developed after the 2009 H1N1 epidemic, the FDA developed RAPID: Real-time Application for Portable Interactive Devices. RAPID is a cloud-based system designed to receive health data, process it, and respond in real time. It was developed based on the experiences of FDA drug safety analysts when they found the need to monitor and evaluate the safety and efficacy of a previously unapproved anti-influenza drug. This drug was provided on an emergency basis to hospitals to treat seriously ill patients who did not respond to traditional therapies, and the FDA was ill-equipped to monitor the safety and efficacy of this drug in real time which in turn inhibited their ability to respond appropriately to the emergency [31].

During the H1N1 epidemic, there was no infrastructure to easily report adverse events data which lead to incomplete and variable quality reports. RAPID is designed to use blockchain based smart contracts to provide real-time, two-way communication between providers and regulators as well as automated event reporting while maintaining compliance with data security and privacy standards. Through the use of RAPID, a provider can submit adverse drug reactions on their mobile device or through their hospital's EHR. These data travel to the FDA and populate a real-time dashboard which enables FDA drug analysts to evaluate and, if necessary, intervene by communicating back to the provider.

Use of blockchain in this case allows for smart contracts that clearly define the data sharing protocols while maintaining the privacy of PHI and PII. This allows for almost completely automatic data sharing which was previously impossible, even in an emergency, due to regulatory constraints. By using smart contracts, the RAPID system can ensure compliance with regulations without any human intervention.

FUTURE DIRECTIONS

Healthcare is undergoing significant changes as it adapts to rising usage and administrative complexity. Health IT is an increasingly large part of that adaption and should, eventually, make healthcare and its administration more transparent and efficient. Blockchain provides a potential solution to many of the issues standing in the way of the promise of health IT. Blockchain makes it easy to establish trust among all the parties in healthcare, facilitates transparent automatic transactions and information distribution and makes auditing the flow of information and money simple. While it's not a silver bullet, the widespread adoption of blockchain in healthcare could help bring about the promise of health IT.

Work remains to be done, however, as blockchain itself has not been fully developed—witness the continuous explosion of new blockchains and platforms built on top of them and full trust in the technology has yet to be established. There are many great ideas out there, but we have yet to see any large-scale adoption and the number of production ready systems is limited. Finally, it is important to remember that for all the promise blockchain holds, it is still just a technology and the economic realities of healthcare are often the true drivers of change.

REFERENCES

1. Nieles, M., Dempsey, K., & Pillitteri, V. Y. (2017). National Institute of Standards and Technology special publication 800-12 Revision 1 CODEN: NSPUE2. *An Introduction to information security.* Retrieved from https://doi.org/10.6028/NIST.SP.800-12r1

2. *Federal Register, 78*(17). Rules and regulations (2013). Retrieved January 25, 2013 from: https://www.gpo.gov/fdsys/pkg/FR-2013-01-25/pdf/2013-01073.pdf

3. Ekblaw, A., Azaria, A., Halamka, J. D., & Lippman, A. (2016). *A case study for blockchain in healthcare: "MedRec" prototype for electronic health records and medical research data.* Azaria, A., Ekblaw, A., Vieira, T., & Lippman, A. (2016). *MedRec: using blockchain for medical data access and permission management* (pp. 25–30). 2nd International Conference on Open and Big Data (OBD), Vienna, 2016, . doi: 10.1109/OBD.2016.11

4. Sullivan, M. T. E. (2017). *Administrative simplification in the physician practice.* Retrieved from https://www.ama-assn.org/sites/default/files/media-browser/public/about-ama/councils/Council%20Reports/council-on-medical-service/i11-cms-administrative-simplification-physician-practice.pdf

5. The Harris Poll. (2012). *Oil, pharmaceutical, health insurance, tobacco, banking and utilities top the list of industries that people would like to see more regulated.* Retrieved from http://www.theharrispoll.com/politics/Oil__Pharmaceutical__Health_Insurance__Tobacco__Banking_and_Utilities_Top_The_List_Of_Industries_That_People_Would_Like_To_See_More_Regulated.html

6. Xu, R. (2015). *The health care industry's relationship problems.* Retrieved from https://www.newyorker.com/business/currency/the-health-care-industrys-relationship-problems

7. Bernstein, L. (2015). *U.S. faces 90,000 doctor shortage by 2025, medical school association warns.* Retrieved from https://www.washingtonpost.com/news/to-your-health/wp/2015/03/03/u-s-faces-90000-doctor-shortage-by-2025-medical-school-association-warns/

8. World Health Organization. (2010). *Health systems financing: The path to universal coverage.* Retrieved from http://www.who.int/whr/2010/en/

9. Evans, R. S. (May 20, 2016). Electronic health records: Then, now, and in the future. *Year Med Inform,* (Suppl 1), S48-61. doi: 10.15265/IYS-2016-s006. Review. PubMed PMID: 27199197; PubMed Central PMCID: PMC5171496.

10. Health Information and the Law. (2016). *Who owns medical records: 50 state comparison.* George Washington University Hirsh Health Law and Policy Program. Retrieved from: http://www.healthinfolaw.org/comparative-analysis/who-owns-medical-records-50-state-comparison

11. U.S. Department of Health and Human Services, Office of Civil Rights (2013).. *HIPAA Administrative Simplification* (45 CFR Parts 160, 162, and 164). Retrieved from http://www.hhs.gov/sites/default/files/hipaa-simplification-201303.pdf

12. Mandl, K. D., Markwell, D., MacDonald, R., Szolovits, P., & Kohane, I. S. (2001). Public standards and patients' control: How to keep electronic medical records accessible but private. *BMJ, 322*(7281), 283–287.

13. Office of the National Coordinator for Health Information Technology. (2015). *Report on health information blocking.* Report to Congress. Retrieved from https://www.healthit.gov/sites/default/files/reports/info_blocking_040915.pdf

14. U.S. Department of Health and Human Services. (2010). *Individuals' right under HIPAA to access their health information* (45 CFR § 164.524). Retrieved 10/31/2019 from https://www.hhs.gov/hipaa/for-professionals/privacy/guidance/access/index.

15. Grossmann, C., Goolsby, W. A., Olsen, L., & McGinnis, J. M. (2010). *Clinical data as the basic staple of health learning: Creating and protecting a public good.* Institute of Medicine of the National Academies Workshop Summary (Learning Health System Series). Washington, DC: National Academies Press.

16. Kish, L. J., & Topol, E. J. (2015). Unpatients—Why patients should own their medical data. *Nature Biotechnology, 33*(9), 921–924.

17. Hayek, F. (n.d.). *The denationalisation of money*—nakamotoinstitute.org. Retrieved from https://nakamotoinstitute.org/static/docs/denationalisation.pdf

18. Dai, W. (1998). *B-money.* Retrieved from http://www.weidai.com/bmoney.txt.

19. Nakamoto, S. (2008). *Bitcoin: A peer-to-peer electronic cash system.* Retrieved 10/31/2019 from: https://bitcoin.org/bitcoin.pdf

20. Ethereum White Paper. (2014). *A next-generation smart contract and decentralized application platform.* Retrieved 10/31/2019 from: https://github.com/ethereum/wiki/wiki/White-Paper

21. Zheng, Z., Xie, S., Dai, H., Chen, X., & Wang, H. (2017). *An overview of blockchain technology: Architecture, consensus, and future trends.* 2017 IEEE International Congress on Big Data (BigData Congress). IEEE (pp. 557–564). doi:10.1109/BigData-Congress.2017.85.

22. Wood, G. (2014). *Ethereum: A secure decentralised generalised transaction ledger. Ethereum project yellow paper, 151,* 1–32. Retrieved from: https://ljk.imag.fr/membres/Jean-Guillaume.Dumas/Enseignements/ProjetsCrypto/Ethereum/ethereum-yellowpaper.pdf

23. Androulaki, E., Barger, A., Bortnikov, V., Cachin, C., ... & Yellick, J. (2018). *Hyperledger fabric: a distributed operating system for permissioned blockchains.* (Article 30). Proceedings of the Thirteenth EuroSys Conference (EuroSys '18). ACM, New York, NY, USA, . DOI: https://doi.org/10.1145/3190508.3190538

24. Madhok, V. (2018). *A foundation of trust for the future of healthcare: An overview of the BItMED Health Protocol.* BitMED Incorporated, BitMED.io Retrieved from

https://github.com/InsighterInc/whitepaper/blob/master/BitMED_Concept_BXMP_v4.pdf

25. Woolhandler, S., Campbell, T., & Himmelstein D. U. (2003). Costs of healthcare administration in the United States and Canada. *N Engl J Med, 349*(8), 768–775. PubMed PMID: 12930930.

26. Sakowski, J. A., Kahn, J. G., Kronick, R. G., Newman, J. M., & Luft, H. S. (2009). Peering into that black box: Billing and insurance activities in a medical group. *Health Affairs, 28*(Supplement 1), w544–w554. Retrieved from https://doi.org/10.1377/hlthaff.28.4.w544

27. Heston, T. F. (2017). A case study in blockchain health care innovation. *International Journal of Current Research, 9*(11), 60587–60588.

28. Einaste, T. (2018). Blockchain and healthcare: The Estonian experience—e-Estonia Retrieved from https://e-estonia.com/blockchain-healthcare-estonian-experience

29. De Meijer, C. R. (2017). *Blockchain in healthcare: Make the industry better* [Internet]. Finextra Research. Retrieved from https://www.finextra.com/blogposting/13801/blockchain-in-healthcare-make-the-industry-better

30. Ekblaw, A., Azaria, A., Halamka, J. D., & Lippman, A. (2016). *A case study for blockchain in healthcare: "MedRec" prototype for electronic health records and medical research data.* Azaria, A., Ekblaw, A., Vieira, T., & Lippman, A. (2016). *MedRec: using blockchain for medical data access and permission management* (pp. 25–30). 2nd International Conference on Open and Big Data (OBD), Vienna, 2016, . doi: 10.1109/OBD.2016.11

31. Francis, H., Jackson, G., Sawarkar, A., Sorbello, A., Walsh, J., & Weaver, B. (2018). *Use of real-time application for portable interactive devices (RAPID) for data safety and patient outcomes.* Silver Spring, MD: US Food and Drug Administration. Retrieved 10/31/2019 from: lexjansen.com/phuse-us/2018/rg/RG11.pdf

CHAPTER 5

HARNESSING THE POWER OF SOCIAL MEDIA ANALYTICS

Atefeh (Anna) Farzinda and Diana Inkpen

INTRODUCTION

Social media is a powerful tool for building community engagement and fostering better relationships with clients. This type of online social experience has revolutionized the healthcare industry, referred to in this domain as "social health." For example, medical forums developed to allow patients to discuss their feelings and experiences, while Twitter enables real-time communication of recommendations, ailments, treatments, and medication for providers and consumers alike.

Social health is not only a discussion-based paradigm. The rise of wearable technologies, such as smart glasses, smart watches, fitness trackers, and sleep monitors also influences social media and communication. Healthcare applications are among the focus areas of wearable technologies. Microsoft, Google, and Apple have released their own health platforms, in which doctors and other health care professionals can monitor the data, text, and voice collected via the patient's wearable technology.

Transforming Healthcare with Big Data and AI, pages 77–89.
Copyright © 2020 by Information Age Publishing
77

NATURAL LANGUAGE PROCESSING (NLP)

The unprecedented volume and variety of user-generated content and the user interaction network constitute new opportunities for understanding social behavior and building socially intelligent health systems. There are several means of interaction in social media platforms. One of the most important is via text posts. The text-rich environment lends itself to a type of machine learning called Natural Language Processing (NLP), which centers around the understanding, prediction, and analysis of large volumes of textual information.

NLP technics enable computers to derive meaning from natural language input using the knowledge from computer science, artificial intelligence, and linguistics. Semantic analysis of social health helps to develop automated tools and algorithms to monitor, capture, and analyze the massive amounts of data collected from social media to predict user health behavior, identify health problem or extract other kinds of information.

SOCIAL MEDIA ONLINE PLATFORMS

Medical forums are among the premier platforms for social health discussion. For example, the popular EHealth forum (ehealthforum.com) is a community site for medical Q&As that offers several subtopics such as mental health, men's and women's health, cancer, relationships, and nutrition. Other sites focus on more specific areas, such as Spine Health (www.spine-health.com), which provides information on back and neck pain relief where members can discuss pain, conditions, and treatment.

The language is often informal; while users may sometimes employ medical terms, most of the time lay language terms are used. Using NLP techniques, various information can be extracted automatically from such forums. In one case, an algorithm may parse the sites to find the appropriate treatment for disc herniation and verify if a lumbar microdiscectomy surgery may be the right solution. In another, the algorithm can find advice on how self-care can help improve back pain via methods such as quitting smoking, exercising, and rehabilitation.

OPINION MINING IN MEDICAL FORUMS

What people think is always an important piece of information. Asking a friend to recommend a dentist or writing a review on a doctor are examples of this importance in our daily life [1]. On social media platforms, such as weblogs, social blogs, microblogging, wikis, and discussion forums, people can easily express and share their opinions. These opinions can be accessed by people who need more information to make decisions. Due to the mass of information exchanged daily on social media, the traditional monitoring techniques are not useful. Therefore, a number of research efforts aim to establish automated tools, which should be intelligent enough to extract the opinion of a writer from a given text.

Processing a text to extract its subjective information is known as sentiment analysis, which is also referred to as opinion mining. The basic goal of sentiment analysis is to identify the overall polarity of a document: positive, negative, or neutral [1]. The polarity magnitude is also taken into account, for example, on a scale of 1 to 5 stars for reviews. Sentiment analysis is not an easy job even for humans, because even two people may disagree on the sentiment expressed in a given text. Therefore, such analysis is a difficult task for the algorithms, and it gets harder when the texts get shorter. Another challenge is to connect the opinion to the entity that is the target of the opinion, and it is often the case that there are multiple aspects of the entities. Users could express positive opinions toward some aspects and negative toward other aspects. For example, a user could like a doctor's office for its location but not for its service quality.

Opinion mining in medical forums is similar to opinion mining in blogs, but the interest is focused on a specific health problem. For example, the study conducted by Tanveer Ali and his colleagues collected texts from medical forums about hearing devices and classified them into negative (e.g., talking about the stigma associated with the wearing of hearing aids), neutral, or positive [2]. A preliminary step is automatic filtering of the posts to keep only those relevant to the topic. Then, for the opinion classification task, the techniques are based on machine learning and counting of polarity terms.

DETECTION OF PERSONAL HEALTH INFORMATION

An important aspect specific to health-related applications is the need for privacy protection. De-identification is the process of removing personal data from documents with sensitive content to protect an individual's privacy from a third party [3][4]. De-identification is very important in health informatics, especially when dealing with patient records. It can be viewed as the detection of personal health information (PHI), such as names, dates of birth, addresses, and health insurance numbers. On social health forums such as Patients Like Me (www.patientslikeme. com), there is a need for detecting PHI and warning the users to revise their postings to protect their confidential personal information.

Detection of PHI on various kinds of text was investigated by Dr. Sokolova and her colleagues [5]. Opinion analysis that considers the detection of sensitive information in Twitter messages about health issues was investigated among others [6]. A somewhat inverse problem to de-identification is to link mentions of the same person across various documents or databases [7], which is critical when one has multiple medical records at different clinics or hospitals.

IDENTIFICATION OF MEDICATION SIDE EFFECTS

Following clinical trials, pharmaceutical researchers rely on patients self-reporting side-effects of prescription medicine. The monitoring of adverse pharmaceutical side effects, known as "pharmacovigilance," has become more accessible to

a) #Schizophrenia*indication* #Seroquel did not suit me at all. Had severe tremors*ADR* and weight gain*ADR*.

b) I felt awful, it made my stomach hurt*ADR* with bad heartburn*ADR* too, horrid taste in my mouth*ADR* tho it does tend to clear up the infection*indication*.

FIGURE 5.1, Examples of annotated social media posts discussing Adverse Drug Reaction [8].

researchers due to the vast amounts of information patients now self-report on social media. An interesting research conducted by Dr. Nikfarjam is into the use of NLP techniques on Adverse Drug Reaction (ADR) extraction from social media [8]. The result was a concept extraction system called ADRMine.

The training of ADRMine relied on two datasets: an expert-annotated corpus of over 8,000 social media posts from Twitter and DailyStrength (a health-focused social network), and an unlabeled corpus of over 1 million user sentences from social media. The researchers learned word embeddings using the latter corpus to generate token similarity information via k-means clustering. This cluster information served as a feature in the final model. Using existing medical language databases, the researchers compiled a lexicon of over 13,000 ADR-related phrases. The ADRMine system's main predictive component was a CRF classifier, trained on the annotated corpus mentioned above.

For features, the researchers used contextual information (the six tokens surrounding the token being classified), a binary feature denoting if the token existed in the ADR phrase lexicon, the token's part-of-speech tag, and a negation tag. Additionally, to improve on baseline performance, the researchers included cluster similarity information, from the k-means clustering mentioned above, on the token being classified and the surrounding context tokens. The final model achieved an evaluation of 0.82 in F-score which could be calculated as:

$$2 \times \frac{\text{precision} \times \text{recall}}{\text{precision} + \text{recall}}.$$

Then, this research is extended to include DeepHealthMiner, a deep learning approach to classifying ADRs, shown in Figure 5.2. This model used over 3 million user sentences to generate word embeddings for tokens. These tokens then served as the input into a feed-forward neural network, which tried to distinguish ADR tokens in a sentence from other types of tokens. Once a token was flagged as an ADR, it was then compared to a lexicon of ADR phrases to predict which ADR the post was discussing. This lexicon-based approach achieved an F-measure of 0.64, lower than that of the ADRMine system.

Other researchers took on the challenging process of extracting ADRs from social media text [10]. Unlike the previous works, these researchers sought to show

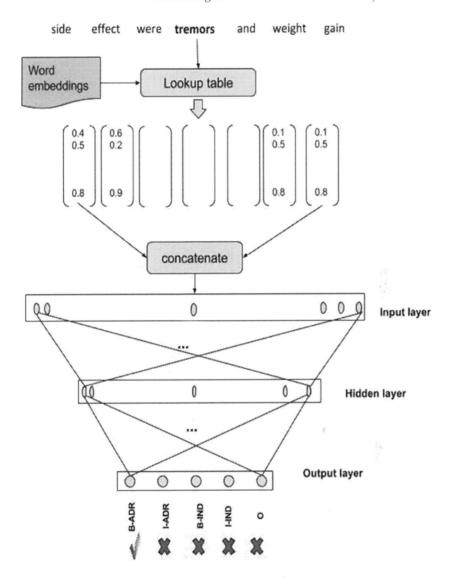

FIGURE 5.2. The DeepHealthMiner Neural Net Architecture [9]

that quality models could be trained without large amounts of expert-annotated training data. Their approach was to develop an active learning system, whereby only a few seed training examples would be needed before the model could start making predictions. A human arbiter would then quickly accept or reject the model's decisions, allowing it to learn without large amounts of expert-labeled data. The central model in this research was a recurrent neural network (RNN), with the input of word embeddings of posts from a social health forum. To augment the word vectorization, the researchers also leveraged DBpedia knowledge graph embeddings, which can provide more useful vectorizations for domain-specific words. This model achieved an F-score of 0.93 when training data was provided and 0.83 when using only active training, thus demonstrating the potential of bootstrapped training when sufficient training data is unavailable.

DETECTION OF MENTAL HEALTH ISSUES

In general, patients tend to post information about their health, the effect of treatments and medication, emotional experiences on social health forums. Data about stress or depressive states could also be useful in detecting potential mental health issues. The discussion of people's mental health has recently grown beyond health-specific forums. For example, some researchers used topic modeling to collect 176 million tweets relating to depression or suicide [11]. Using this dataset, the researchers analyzed communication patterns in users discussing these mental health issues. Such research could prove useful in improving the logistics and organization of mental health outreach campaigns on social media platforms.

With the increase in social media usage and the extensive level of self-disclosure [12], more and more research has been conducted to identify mental disorders at an individual as well as at a society level. Researchers have used features such as behavioral characteristics, depression language, emotion, and linguistic style, reduced social activity, increased negative effects, clustered social networks, raised interpersonal and medical fears, increased expression in religious involvement, and use of negative words to determine the cues of major depressive disorder [13]. In addition, syntactical features such as bag of words (BOW) and word frequencies are used to identify the ratio of tweet topics, concluding that topic modeling also adds a positive contribution to the predictive model compared to the use of the BOW model, which could also result in overfitting [14].

The successful use of NLP techniques in identifying the progress and level of depression of individuals in online therapy could bring greater insights to clinicians, assisting them in applying interventions effectively and efficiently. In another interesting study, 882 transcripts gathered from an online psychological therapy provider to determined that use of linguistic features can be considered as more valuable in predicting the progress of a patient compared to sentiment and topic-based analysis [15]. Contrary to traditional sentiment analysis approaches that use three main polarity classes (i.e., positive, negative, and neutral), Shickel and Rashidi divided the neutral class into two classes: neither positive nor negative and both positive and negative [16]. With the use of syntactic, lexical, and by representing words as vectors in the vector space (word embeddings), the authors managed to achieve an overall accuracy of 78% for the four-class polarity prediction.

A Microsoft research proposed methods to identify the level of depression among social media users including automatic calculations of a social media depression (SMDI: Social Media Depression Index) [17]. Another recent study used a classification model trained with n-grams, linguistic behavior and Latent Dirichlet Allocation (LDA) topics as features for predicting the individuals who are susceptible to having depression [18]. Many researchers used open-vocabulary analysis and lexicon-based approaches such as Linguistic Inquiry and Word Count (LIWC), which is a text analysis software that calculates the degree of use for different categories of words across a wide array of texts [19]. In addition to that, the use of language models is proposed to determine the existence of mental disorders [20]. Language models are based on unigrams and character 5-grams which provides context to distinguish between words and phrases that sound similar.

The Computational Linguistics and Clinical Psychology (CLPsych) 2015 shared task [21] used self-reported data on Twitter about Post Traumatic Stress Disorder (PTSD) and depression, collected according to the procedure introduced by Coppersmith, Dredze and Harman in the previous year [22]. The shared task participants were provided with a dataset of self-reported users on PTSD and depression. For each user in the dataset, nearly 3,200 recent posts were collected using the Twitter API. The system which was ranked first in the CLPsych 2015 Shared Task, created 16 systems based on features derived using supervised LDA, supervised anchors (for topic modeling), lexical TF-IDF, and a combination of all [23]. An SVM classifier with a linear kernel obtained an average precision above 0.80 for all the three tasks (i.e., depression vs. control, PTSD vs. control and depression vs. PTSD) and a maximum precision of 0.893 for differentiating PTSD users from the control group. Another system employed user metadata and textual features from the corpus provided by the CLPsych 2015 Shared Task to develop a linear classifier to predict users having either one of the mental illnesses [24]. They used the BOW approach to aggregate word counts, topics derived from clustering methods and metadata (e.g., followers, followees, age, gender) from the users Twitter profile as the main feature categories. With the use of logistic regression and linear SVM in an ensemble of classifiers, the authors managed to obtain an average precision above 0.800 for all the three tasks and with a maximum score of 0.867 for differentiating users in the control group from the users with depression.

The use of the supervised LDA and the supervised anchor model was proven to be highly successful compared to the unsupervised clustering approaches, and even more efficient than using linguistic methods such as the use of n-grams and other lexicon-based approaches. Such approaches can be successfully used in identifying users with depression, who have self-disclosed their mental illnesses on Twitter [23]. In general, a clear distinction in the lexical and syntactic structure of the language used by individuals with different mental disorders, as well as between individuals within a control group, can be identified throughout the literature mentioned above, as well as from the explorative analysis [25].

The novel method introduced by Coppersmith leverages self-diagnoses posted on Twitter to identify users with mental health conditions [26]. They expanded this research to include results for ten different conditions and to control for gender and age demographics. The data collection process involved scanning through posts on Twitter for statements such as "I have just been diagnosed with X" where X matched one of the ten conditions being examined. For each diagnosed user, over 100 tweets were collected.

To discriminate between conditions, the researchers examined differences in LIWC categories between users with various conditions. Such analysis demonstrated that certain conditions (e.g., eating disorder and seasonal affective disorder) display distinct linguistic patterns, while others (e.g., anxiety and depression) are harder to distinguish. To broaden the vocabulary used in this discrimination, the researchers included use of character-based n-gram models (CLMs). Using CLM scores for each condition achieved high accuracy in discrimination for particular conditions (86% accuracy for anxiety, 76% accuracy for eating disorders). This suggests that using linguistic features for mental health condition discrimination could prove fruitful moving forward.

A recent study leveraged the datasets from the above research [26] to design a novel neural architecture for mental health diagnoses through Twitter [27]. Using three datasets identifying Twitter users as belonging to a specific set of mental health disorders, the researchers trained a multi-task learning (MLT) model that shared parameters of three independently trained neural nets. They hypothesized that the patterns expressed in the three datasets would be highly correlated, and thus good candidates for MLT. The results of these experiments varied across disease classification but demonstrated significant improvements in the bipolar disorder and post-traumatic stress disorder (PTSD) tasks, which had the least training data.

The researchers from the University of Ottawa proposed an automated system that can identify at-risk users from their public social media activity, more specifically, from Twitter [28]. The data was collected is from the #BellLetsTalk campaign, which is a wide-reaching, multi-year program designed to break the silence around mental illness and support mental health across Canada. The annotated dataset included 160 users. The researchers trained a user-level classifier for detecting at-risk users. They also trained a tweet-level classifier for predicting if a tweet indicates depression. This task was much more difficult due to the imbalanced data (in average, there were about 5% depression tweets and 95% non-depression tweets per depressed user) and to the lack of information in a short tweet.

To handle the class imbalance, undersampling methods were used. The resulting classifier at tweet-level had high recall, but low precision. Therefore, this classifier was only used to compute the estimated percentage of depressed tweets and to add this value as a feature for the user-level classifier. The best results for the user-level classification on the #BellLetsTalk dataset were 0.70 precision, 0.85 recall and 0.77 F-score for an SVM classifier with features such as polarity word counts, depression word counts, and the number of pronouns, plus the automatically estimated percentage of depressed tweets for each user.

Deep Learning technique was also used for detecting signs of depression [29]. They testes various architectures (CNN, RNN) and various kinds of word embedding (readily available and specially trained on a depression corpus). They trained the classifiers on part of CLPsych 2015 dataset and tested on a set-aside part of the same dataset. In addition, they tested on the #BellLetsTalk dataset mentioned above [28] to show that the models are generalizable. Their experiments showed that the CNN-based models perform better than RNN-based models. Models with optimized embeddings managed to maintain performance with the generalization ability.

The task of identifying posts discussing mental health and discerning what specific conditions are being discussed has been a primary focus of social media health research. Gkotsis and his colleagues took such a linguistic approach to analyze mental health posts on the popular social media forum Reddit, which provides many topic-specific forums called "subreddits" [25]. In this study, the task was to determine which linguistic features could be useful in identifying posts related to mental health conditions and other applications such as identifying posts requiring urgent attention.

The researchers collected posts from 16 subreddits dedicated to the discussion of ten different mental health conditions. The feature set from these texts included measures established from previous psycholinguistic work, such as LIWC and Coh-Metrix, and different measures of readability and complexity. To examine complexity, the researchers used features such as cohesion (measured in word overlap between sentences), horizontal complexity (measured in sentence count), and vertical complexity (measured in the height of the parse tree for each sentence).

The results indicated that there is not much linguistic variance between subreddits, meaning that such features would not be sufficient for classification systems. However, by comparing the differences in vocabularies across mental health discussions, the researchers were able to note significant similarities (60% accuracy in discrimination) between subreddits dedicated to the same condition and differences (90% accuracy in discrimination) between those dedicated to different conditions.

SHARED TASKS ON CLINICAL PSYCHOLOGY DATABASE

The shared task at CLPsych 2016 and 2017 further challenge the research community in the task of developing classifiers to automatically prioritize posts from an online peer-support forum for youth mental health and wellbeing hosted by ReachOut.com. These forums are carefully moderated by a team of trained professionals and volunteers, who ensure they remain safe, positive and healthy. The shared task aims to support these moderators by automatically identifying concerning content so that it can be addressed as quickly as possible.

For this task, ReachOut has annotated a corpus of posts with a red/amber/green semaphore that indicates how urgently they require moderator attention. Systems leveraged the content of the posts, including sentiment, topics, thread context, and user history, to classify posts into the three classes: red, amber, or green. A fourth class, named crisis, is also available, with very few training instances. Posts labeled as crisis require the urgent intervention of the moderators. In addition to the 947 training posts, a separate set of 241 test posts were annotated for use in the evaluation of the shared task systems. Some of the best results in the 2016 shared task were obtained by Shickel and Rashidi, who used normalized unigrams in conjunction with a broader range of post features, with some attributes based on the number and content of other posts in the same thread [16]. Their system achieved average precision, recall, and F-measure of 0.84, 0.83, and 0.82, respectively. Brew demonstrated green precision, recall, and F-measure of 0.93, 0.84, and 0.88 respectively, with better differentiation between amber and red posts [30]. Brew's system used a small feature set and emphasized the use of a SMO classifier with radial kernel. The 2017 shared task used the data from 2016, plus a new test set and the possibility to use additional unlabeled data.

CONCLUSION

Over time, social media has become a part of common healthcare. The healthcare industry uses social media tools for building community engagement and fostering better relationships with their clients. In this chapter, we have demonstrated some of the applications for social media analysis in healthcare that require natural language processing and semantic analysis of textual social data. Social media analyzing applications are increasingly in demand with the growth of social media data and user-generated content in various platforms. There are many challenges in understanding large social media data environments, including architecture, security, integrity, management, scalability, artificial intelligence, NLP techniques, distribution, and visualization.

Health informatics is a new and rapidly growing interdisciplinary field addressing the development of automated tools and algorithms. NLP techniques in social health have revolutionized the field and improved the provider workflow and patient care by monitoring, capturing, and analyzing big data collected from social networks. In the future, the rapid advancement of technology will change the way humans and machines operate. In this chapter, we highlighted the relevant NLP tools for social media data with the purpose of integrating them into real-world applications by reviewing the latest in NLP innovative methods for social media analysis.

REFERENCES

1.   Pang, B., & Lee, L. (2018). Opinion mining and sentiment analysis. *Foundations and trends in Information Retrieval, 2*(1–2), 135, 2008.

2. Ali, T., Schramm, D., Sokolova, M., & Inkpen, D. (2013). Can I hear you? Opinion learning from medical forums. *Proceedings of the 6th International Joint Conference on Natural Language Processing.* Retrieved from: http://www.aclweb.org/anthology/I13-1077.

3. Uzuner, Ö., Luo, Y., & Szolovits, P. (2007). Evaluating the state-of-the-art in automatic de-identification. *Journal of the American Medical Informatics Association, 14* (5), 550–563.

4. Yeniterzi, R., Aberdeen, J., Bayer, S., Wellner, B., Hirschman, L., & Malin, B. (2010). Effects of personal identifier resynthesis on clinical text de-identification. *Journal of the American Medical Informatics Association, 17*(2), 159–168.

5. Sokolova, M., El Emam, K., Rose, S., Chowdhury, S., Neri, E., Jonker, E., & Peyton, L. (2009). Personal health information leak prevention in heterogeneous texts. *Proceedings of the workshop on adaptation of language resources and technology to new domains* (pp. 58–69). ACL URL http://dl.acm.org/citation.cfm?id=1859148.1859157.

6. Bobicev, V., Sokolova, M.,Jafer, Y., & Schramm, D. (2012). Learning sentiments from tweets with personal health information. In *Advances in artificial intelligence* (pp. 37–48). Berlin: Springer, URL http://dx.doi.org/10.1007/978-3-642-30353-1_4.

7. Ruths, D., & Liu, W. (2013). *AAAI Spring Symposium: Analyzing microtext.* AAAI, URL http://dblp.uni-trier.de/db/conf/aaaiss/aaaiss2013-01.html#LiuR13.

8. Nikfarjam, A., Sarker, A., O'Connor, K., Ginn, R., & Gonzalez, G. (2015). Pharmacovigilance from social media: Mining adverse drug reaction mentions using sequence labeling with word embedding cluster features. *Journal of the American Medical Informatics Association, 22*(3), 671–681.

9. Nikfarjam, A. (2016). *Health information extraction from social media.* PhD thesis, Arizona State University, URL http://gradworks.umi.com/10/14/10146991.html.

10. Stanovsky, G., Gruhl, D., & Mendes, P. N. (2017). Recognizing mentions of adverse drug reaction in social media using knowledge-infused recurrent models. *Proceedings of the 15th Conference of the European Chapter of the Association for Computational Linguistics: Volume 1, Long Papers* (pp. 142–151). Valencia, Spain: Association for Computational Linguistics. URL http://www.aclweb.org/anthology/E17-1014.

11. McClellan, C., Ali, M. M., Mutter, R., Kroutil, L., & Landwehr, J. (2017). Using social media to monitor mental health discussions—Evidence from twitter. *Journal of the American Medical Informatics Association.* Retrieved from: https://academic.oup.com/jamia/article/24/3/496/2907899; doi: 10.1093/jamia/ocw133

12. Park, M., Cha, C., & Cha, M. (2012). *Depressive moods of users portrayed in Twitter* (pp. 1–8). ACM SIGKDD Workshop on Healthcare Informatics (HI-KDD). ISBN 9781450315487.

13. De Choudhury, M., Counts, S., & Horvitz, E. (2013a). *Social media as a measurement tool of depression in populations* (pp. 47–56). Retrived from: http://dl.acm.org/citation.cfm?doid=2464464.2464480{\%}5Cnpapers3://publication/doi/10.1145/2464464.2464480.

14. Tsugawa, S., Kikuchi, Y., Kishino, F., Nakajima, K., Itoh, Y., & Ohsaki, H. (2015). *Recognizing depression from Twitter activity.* Retrieved from 33rd Annual ACM Conference on Human Factors in Computing Systems—CHI '15, pages 3187–3196, ISBN 9781450331456. doi: 10.1145/2702123.2702280: http://dl.acm.org/citation.cfm?doid=2702123.2702280

15. Howes, C., Purver, M., & McCabe, R. (2014). *Linguistic indicators of severity and progress in online text-based therapy for depression* (pp. 7–16). Workshop on Computational Linguistics and Clinical Psychology, number 611733. ISBN 978-1-941643-16-7.

16. Shickel, B., & Rashidi, P. (2016). *Automatic triage of mental health forum posts.* Retrieved from Proceedings of the Third Workshop on Computational Linguistics and Clinical Psychology (pp. 188–192), San Diego, CA, USA. Association for Computational Linguistics: http://www.aclweb.org/anthology/W16-0326

17. De Choudhury, M., Gamon, M., Counts, S., & Horvitz, E. (2013b). *Predicting depression via social media.* Retrieved from Proceedings of the Seventh International AAAI Conference on Weblogs and Social Media (volume 2, pp. 128–137). ISBN 9781450313315: http://www.aaai.org/ocs/index.php/ICWSM/ICWSM13/paper/viewFile/6124/6351

18. Schwartz, H. A., Eichstaedt, J., Kern, M. L., Park, G., Sap, M., , Stillwell, D., Kosinski M., & Ungar, L. (2014). *Towards assessing changes in degree of depression through Facebook.* Retrieved from Proceedings of the Workshop on Computational Linguistics and Clinical Psychology: From Linguistic Signal to Clinical Reality (pp. 118–125). Retrieved from: http://www.aclweb.org/anthology/W/W14/W14-3214

19. Pennebaker, J. W., Booth, R. J., & Francis, M. E. (2007). *Operator's manual: Linguistic inquiry and word count* (LIWC2007). Technical report, Austin, Texas, LIWC.net, .

20. Coppersmith, G., Dredze, M., & Craig Harman (2014a). Measuring Post Traumatic Stress Disorder in Twitter. *Proceedings of the 7th International AAAI Conference on Weblogs and Social Media (ICWSM)* (volume 2, pp. 23–45). AAAI.

21. Coppersmith, G., Dredze, M., Harman, C., Hollingshead, K., & Mitchell, M. (2015b). CLPsych 2015 shared task: Depression and PTSD on Twitter. In *Proceedings of the 2nd Workshop on Computational Linguistics and Clinical Psychology: From Linguistic Signal to Clinical Reality* (pp. 31–39). doi: 10.3115/v1/w15-1204.

22. Coppersmith, G., Dredze, M., & Harman, C. (2014b). *Quantifying mental health signals in Twitter.* Retrieved from Proceedings of the Workshop on Computational Linguistics and Clinical Psychology: From Linguistic Signal to Clinical Reality (pp. 51–60). Retrieved from: http://www.aclweb.org/anthology/W/W14/W14-3207

23. Resnik, P., Armstrong, W., Claudino, L., Nguyen, T., Nguyen V., & Boyd-Graber, J. (2015). Beyond LDA : Exploring supervised topic modeling for depression-related language in Twitter. In *Proceedings of the 2nd Workshop on Computational Linguistics and Clinical Psychology: From Linguistic Signal to Clinical Reality, volume 1* (pp. 99–107). Denver, CO. Retrieved from: https://www.aclweb.org/anthology/W15-1212/

24. Preotiuc-Pietro, D., Sap, M., Schwartz, H. A., & Ungar, L. (2015a). Mental illness detection at the world well-being project for the CLPsych 2015 Shared Task. *Proceedings of the 2nd Workshop on Computational Linguistics and Clinical Psychology: From Linguistic Signal to Clinical Reality*, (pp. 40–45). Denver, CO. Retrieved from: https://www.aclweb.org/anthology/volumes/W15-12/

25. Gkotsis, G., Oellrich, A., Hubbard, T. J. P., Dobson, R. J. B., Liakata, M., Velupillai S., & Dutta, R. (2016). The language of mental health problems in social media. *Proceedings of the third workshop on computational linguistics and clinical psychology* (pp. 63–73). San Diego, CA, USA: Association for Computational Linguistics.

26. Coppersmith, G., Dredze, M., Harman, C., & Hollingshead, K.. (2015a). *From ADHD to SAD: Analyzing the language of mental health on twitter through self-reported diagnoses.* In *Proceedings of the 2nd workshop on computational linguistics and clinical psychology: From linguistic signal to clinical reality* (pp. 1–10). Denver, CO: Association for Computational Linguistics. Retrieved from: http://www.aclweb.org/anthology/W15-1201

27. Benton, A., Mitchell, M., & Hovy, D. (2017). Multitask learning for mental health conditions with limited social media data. *Proceedings of the 15th conference of the european chapter of the association for computational linguistics* (Volume 1, Long Papers, pp. 152–162). Valencia, Spain: Association for Computational Linguistics. Retrieved from: http://www.aclweb.org/anthology/E17-1015

28. Jamil, Z., Inkpen, D., Buddhitha, P., & White K. (2017). Monitoring tweets for depression to detect at-risk users. *Proceedings of the fourth workshop on computational linguistics and clinical psychology—from linguistic signal to clinical reality* (pp. 32–40). Vancouver, BC. Association for Computational Linguistics. Retrieved from: http://www.aclweb.org/anthology/W17-3104

29. Orabi, A. H., Buddhitha, P., Orabi, M. H., & Inkpen, D. (2018). *Deep learning for depression detection of Twitter users.* Computational Linguistics and Clinical Psychology Workshop CLPsych 2018 at NAACL 2018 New Orleans, LA

30. Brew, C. (2016). Classifying reachout posts with a radial basis function svm. *Proceedings of the third workshop on computational linguistics and clinical psychology* (pp. 138–142). San Diego, CA: Association for Computational Linguistics. Retrieved from: http://www.aclweb.org/anthology/W16-0315

CHAPTER 6

ENHANCING HEALTHCARE DECISION-MAKING WITH DATA-DRIVEN METHODS AND TECHNOLOGY

Alexandra C. Ehrlich

INTRODUCTION

The last 30 years have been an exciting time in healthcare analytics. The pace of data collection and data storage technology has surpassed our ability to come up with ways to use the data and technology tools to help us. In present day we are dealing with a different set of challenges. We are on pace to collect 44 trillion gigabytes by 2020 across different types and as new data collection mediums are born [1]. This information can be used for operations, billing, research, and many other lines of business and perspectives within a healthcare setting. This information can also create secondary value in aggregate by showing trends, correlations and other information useful for other patients in the system.

Each day our systems collect large amounts of data from our patients, providers and payors. Our justification for collection and storing personal and health data is that the data will provide ample benefit for the parties that are both providing and collecting the data. This creates financial implications as well as social

Transforming Healthcare with Big Data and AI, pages 91–104.

91

implications that have guided recommendations and best practices how this data is handled and used. At the center of this paradigm is the patient who, as they go through a system, generate information at each touch point. And at the heart of all these advancements is the aim of maximizing both our financial and social investment. How do we take disparate data points and harness the power of the aggregate to answer more complex questions?

We are currently at the verge of what we can call tertiary use of the data. Utilizing streaming data, metadata, learning systems and other novel technologies to further advance our insights. We are asking new questions and combining new perspectives to innovate and increase value. How do we translate data into action? How do we get buy-in from the stakeholders? How do we fulfill our responsibility to create value and benefit for all those involved?

Below we present a 3-point model for successful insight generation analytics. This model describes the essential qualities to execute a successful analytic plan, large or small. It also shows the interplay of all the pivotal points involved in analytics and the co-dependencies of the analytic process.

Data: the raw material of any analytics plan is the data we must work with. It creates the context, the depth and the usefulness of the insight generated. The data also defines what questions we can ask and who the insights will apply to.

Technology: technology influences what data we receive, in what format, and the level of analytic prowess we can apply to its analysis. This can often become the bottleneck in the process of analysis as data is being collected faster each day and technologies tend lagging in both development and adoption.

Expertise: this is the human capital behind analytics. The end user, the data collector, the business consumer, the patient. Regardless of data or technology, the definition of a successful analytic project depends on how much trust, buy-in and usefulness the stakeholders find in the insight generated.

The three points of the triangle intercept and create a shape and a context for a project large or small. It also creates transparency, traceability and establishes trust in both the insight generated.

We will explore each component, the challenges and opportunities and how they influence insight generation. Addressing our present status as well as the history and process of advancement in data driven healthcare insight generation is pivotal holistically looking towards the future. It is important to note that these are all actionable points in the process. While there are external influences that affect an organization, we will concentrate on what is actionable and what an institution can control, plan and address to mitigate for external influences.

A successful analytics model is shown in Figure 6.1:

Project failure can be traced back to a gap in addressing one or more of the components in the model. Below are some of the common failure points:

- Data: projects that fail to vet, clean and create transparency in the data acquisition or analytic process.

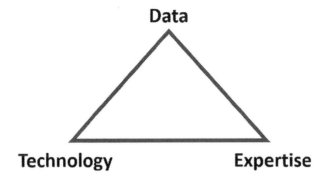

FIGURE 6.1. A Successful Analytics Model

- Technology: projects that use outdated technology or technology that burdens the end user.
- Expertise: projects that do not include subject matter or business user insight.

THE RAW MATERIALS: DATA AND DATA COLLECTION

Let's begin with the simplest question: why do we collect healthcare data? There are 2 reasons why we collect information: direct benefit such as clinical care and billing or assumed future value for better patient outcomes, system improvement and longitudinal and historical patient information. This means that there are two types of data collected and systems associated with that collection. Data that is purpose specific and data that is collected generically for future use. This distinction is important to make from the start as it has a trickledown effect across the continuum of analysis.

Data is collected at every single point of contact in a healthcare encounter. The encounter begins long before the patient becomes a "patient" in a traditional sense. The data collection begins at first contact. A phone call to schedule a visit sets off a cascade of information gathering. If we think of our experience in this scenario, we can think of a simple phone call to schedule a yearly checkup exam. Our name and address are collected (personal information), our insurance details (payor), the reason for our scheduled visit (billing), our preferred or available physician, nurse or PA (provider) and a date and time of appointment (scheduling block). This is all information that we have provided and has been captured before we walk in through the door of a healthcare facility.

Once a patient enters through the doors there is exponential growth in both the data volume and the sensitivity of the data. We fill out health history, family history and, questionnaires while in the waiting room. Vitals, biometrics, concerns, with the nurse at intake and then examination information, labs, prescriptions, treatment plan, with the physician. By the time you are checking out the system collects out of pocket costs and follow up appointment information. This single event or encounter has amassed significant data points that can and will be used in a variety of ways as they relate to the event (primary use) and potentially in the aggregate (secondary use).

This example illustrates the burden of data collection and data protection on the patient and the system in a simple medical encounter. This chapter will explore the challenges and opportunities of generating the raw material of analytics, data.

Challenges

Disparate Data

As described in the chapter introduction, data is collected at different points of the healthcare continuum. This data is collected by a variety of tools, systems and users. The data is in different formats and different levels of complexity. Truly impactful healthcare analytics often leverage data across systems to connect to a larger context to generate insight on patient history, experience and outcomes. This is complex to conceptualize and execute efficiently in our current insight generation models. This challenge has been the central focus of most of the IT investment in the past decades. In previous decades there was large investment in the data collection efforts. That investment and the efforts were effective and have now shifted our focus on connecting the dots across data collecting systems.

While technology and systems have been a focus of the disconnected nature of data, another culprit has been data mandates such as security requirements. Internal protocols and data mandates are often barriers in connecting disparate data systems. These types of protocols are often created for data protection and are rarely revised as the information ecosystems evolves. This can become a barrier and a bottleneck as organizational needs and expectations change. While we have made strides towards improving connection across siloed systems through technology and internal mandates and protocols this remains one of the basic challenges in fully realizing the potential of data in healthcare.

Data Volume

We collect vast amounts of data related to clinical event (patient symptoms, current medications, etc.) and the metadata that gives context to the data collected (time stamps, signature trail). Data from monitors and streaming devices also generate a vast number of records. The challenge lies in that currently, systems that are built to handle large data volumes are built for archiving purposes. These systems lack the nimbleness to surface the data to analysis tools and user interfaces or enable analytic methods that require on demand data or real time data. The biggest challenge in data volume is capturing data that we may not know how we will use but we know is important. This requires some forward thinking and investments without an articulated ROI.

This also requires the use of novel approaches to data storage that often mean hybrid approaches that are specific to the organization and where there may not be off the shelf technology or best practices readily applicable. Addressing the specific infrastructure needed to handle data volume is more of an artform than a science. Along with data volume, we have the complexity of the data to consider. The challenges of data remaining meaningful to a variety of downstream users and perspectives a key consideration. Also, data storage that enables a large portfolio of downstream applications and empowers a variety of users. Decisions made as we consider the solutions to handle the data volume within an institution heavily influence downstream capabilities.

Data Systems

Traditional systems are adept at data storage but have become taxed as more of that data needs to be surfaced to a variety of end users and tools. Traditional infrastructure may create silos and exclude some novel data types. The current challenge is to modernize healthcare systems to be flexible to the ongoing changes and demands of insight generation. Another challenge in the modernization of data systems and infrastructure is the competing priorities of IT investment within an organization. The last decade saw budgets stretched to an extreme as organizations of different sizes implemented electronic medical/health records. These implementations are arguably some of the largest, most complex projects impacting every part of healthcare: patients, providers, resources and IT we have undertaken in the last 30 years.

In the aftermath of these implementations we are challenged to make further IT investment within burdened systems to maximize the realization of value across the enterprise. In the new wave of creating value there is a need to articulate added benefit of further investment as well as convincing leadership and users alike of the added downstream worth of potentially disruptive, albeit temporary, activities.

Data Collection

Traditionally, data in healthcare has been collected for reimbursement and billing purposes. As our analytic capabilities and the culture of healthcare began to shift into a patient-centered model the questions we have asked of the data have evolved but the systems and technology to collect and analyze the data have lagged. This is currently challenging the healthcare system to seek adequate methods to analyze data, efficient technology and tools, and most importantly processes for data collection plans, data security and data access.

Data collection, data storage, data utilization and data security have a delicate interplay in healthcare. The secondary and downstream use of healthcare data is riddled with both technical and consent issues that need to be addressed. The challenge in modernizing the system to enable insight generation is a delicate one. Balancing the components above is the ongoing challenge in most institutions. There is no single answer and organizations often need to experiment with a variety of approaches to find a good fit specific to their goals, funding, and expectations.

Data Integrity

The complexity of our current healthcare model results in data that is generally disorganized and siloed. We have a technologically fractured system that collects data that is often detached from key contextual information. The integrity of this data for its intended use and other downstream use is an important challenge to tackle. While most organizations have made progress on this front, many of the systems in healthcare are still antiquated. The continued use of these systems can be driven by legacy requirements, user preference or specific use cases, such as registries or reporting mandates. Regardless of the reasons behind the use of non-optimal systems that may compromise data integrity, they are a persistent challenge for enterprise use of data and the data integrity requisite for successful analytics.

As the systems modernize and the questions become more complex and ask more of the data collected, there is a need to increase the rigor of how we handle data. Data integrity is a layered process of tracking data from data entry point through analytic consumption. Data integrity provides an important component of insightful and useful analytics, trust. This will remain a challenge in healthcare due to the ongoing changes in systems, sources and technology. As a persistent consideration it must be revised and revisited often to optimize.

Data Standardization

There are two key components in the process of data standardization. The technical side involves creating an ecosystem of data collection and storage tools that can be connected. The systems must be flexible and nimble to adapt to changing needs. The other component is using standard language, terminologies and other standards across the enterprise that are industry vetted and centrally maintained. This upfront work is all about long term maintenance and support of the system. While it is hard to predict future needs, standardization will create a supported context and framework as the needs evolve.

Accomplishing data standardization is both an internal and external challenge. Internally, it impacts the variety of use cases that can leverage certain data, therefore impacting the full realization of value of the data. Externally, lack of standards creates a bottleneck on data sharing that may impede advancements from research collaborations to patient-centric care goals. While there are several standards for both terminologies as well as electronic data sharing, healthcare organizations have been slow in adoption as there is little consensus on how and to which standards to align to. Future breakthroughs in this area will create exponential benefit to internal and external systems and will have a great impact on healthcare and all stakeholders.

Opportunities

Security

Addressing security within a healthcare institution will most likely always remain in the "opportunities" category. Threats to data security change and evolve daily and systems will need to stay vigilant to stay a step ahead of the threats. Data mandates also evolve swiftly, and the responsibility and burden will remain on the institutions to stay compliant through processes, methods and technology. Securing data will remain the highest priority as this is the most basic IT endeavor that will become either a bottleneck or an opportunity to grow trust in the system and therefore open more doors for analytics, collaborations and other undertakings that help realize the value and promise of data. Security is an area where remaining on the cutting edge and leveraging new technologies and methods is imperative.

The opportunities here are vast. The variety of approaches, technology and vendors in this space may be overwhelming but the key benefit in this variety is that there is an imperative to continued innovation and investment to security, especially as healthcare data volumes grow. Another opportunity creates systems that enable patient-controlled permissions, such as the new approaches control and access in the European Union, where patients have more control of the information that is retained and shared as individuals. This is not a trivial undertaking from a system or technology perspective. We can pave the way to more efficient systems and approaches as more contextual data becomes part of patient's care (activity monitor, Internet of Things, etc.)

Patient Voice

The patient voice is becoming a central tenant of how we measure healthcare outcomes. While the last decade saw a move towards the patient centric model of care, data collection for the patient perspective has continue to use non-optimal methods. We have been leveraging surveys to capture the patient reported experience for decades. And while survey methodology now leverages novel technology there are other innovative technology approaches, such as "smart rooms" that consume data from monitors and sensors surrounding the patient during an encounter to validate and add context to patient reported data.

The concept of patient experience and the inception of the Chief Experience Officer (CXO) is an exciting attempt to begin to truly put the patient voice at the center of how we design care systems. Healthcare institutions are investing in monitors, devices and other Internet of Things (IoT) methods to capture real time information about patient flow, interactions and experience. This is a promising area that is taking experience from other fields such as hospitality and retail and attempting to translate best practices into real world protocols that resonate in a healthcare setting.

As this is a field in its infancy, we are encountering some of the usual challenges. A deluge of data is coming in and the system imperative is to make sense of it. The technology to collect the data has evolved yet our systems to process and gain insight are still lacking. Some of the novel approaches of big data and artificial intelligence are now and will remain central approaches in finding creative solutions for insight generation. Capturing the patient voice is a great opportunity to innovate and bring value to our central stakeholder, the patient.

Provider Experience

In the last five years the provider voice has become a prevalent perspective of interest. Although the provider voice has always been part of the decision-making process when it comes to analytics, the growing complexity of use cases and technology have created a need for a more efficient way to track and capture provider information. We are seeing large numbers of providers (nurses, doctors, etc.) becoming fatigued by both the system demands and the technology associated with those systems. Technology and workflow changes often impact the delivery of care and creates demands on already strained human resources.

The opportunity here lies in including the provider voice early in the process of technology decision making and creating systems that encourage user adoption. IT decisions are often made without the provider buy-in and insight. Without provider insight the data collected is often used to create metrics that can have a punitive connotation. This can create a difficult culture and become a barrier for user adoption of both technology and use of insights generated by the system.

Understanding and including the provider voice early in the process of analytics insight generation projects is a great opportunity to build trust and ownership. A strong IT and provider partnership are crucial to successful analytic endeavors (Expertise component). This will not only improve the provider experience, retention and performance but through compliance to the systems and protocols we will see improved data downstream. This will create a trickle-down effect that impacts actionable healthcare insight and fosters an environment where innovation and technology can save lives.

Novel Data

Novel data is increasing both the potential and the complexity of systems and analytics. Data coming from a variety of non-traditional sources is creating a new phase in our healthcare insight journey and the promise of the actionable insights we may generate from it. Often unstructured, novel data can come from medical or commercial devices that track patient behavior patterns. It can be sourced from sensors that track workflows such as drug dispensing and resource efficiency. Novel data also encompasses aggregate and processed data generated by machine learning or artificial intelligence processes that can add context to traditional data.

Our greatest opportunity in this area is in the creation of infrastructure that supports new data types and enables us to leverage the complexity to answer advanced questions. Creating a culture of innovation that is open to new perspectives and embraces the complexity of novel data types from the ground up will be pivotal in realizing the full benefits this data can bring to healthcare insights. It is also pivotal to differentiate innovation from daily requirements and create systems that support discovery while maintaining solid infrastructure for tried and tested methods.

All the opportunities in the data area have a common thread. A call to create flexible systems that scale and adapt and to become comfortable with the ambiguity of the unknown of technology developments and the shifting demands of healthcare. These are difficult concepts to apply in healthcare settings where the data mandates and responsibilities to protect the data are pivotal and prioritized above any other analytic endeavor. This requires a sensitive culture shifting approach that impacts both healthcare providers and the technology developers. We must move away from the reactive model of technology deployment and proactively and creatively finding solutions that maximize what we can do today and mitigate for the unknown requirements of the future.

The opportunities and challenges of the data component are to enhance decision making by creating a solid foundation and creating trust as the complexity of systems increases. Data is the building block of any insight generating analytic process. This is where we build trust, variety and innovation. By enhancing the building blocks of analytics, we cultivate for future breakthroughs in healthcare.

THE TOOLS: TECHNOLOGY AND HUMAN CAPITAL

As we have explored earlier, one of the biggest challenges in healthcare data analytics the last decade has been data handling as more and more sources generate more information. If data is the raw material, the next step in the process of generating actionable insights requires tools, methods and human capital to transform data. Large data volumes and types of data, coupled with the pace of change in mandates and expectations in healthcare data downstream tools, methods and experts need to remain flexible and current. Below we will explore the challenges and opportunities and the key factors that make up our toolbox for actionable insight generation.

Challenges

Tools

Along with the deluge of data, the last decades have seen an equivalent deluge of tools that aim to wrangle, analyze and surface the data. There are 3 common approaches in the development of tools/deployment of analytic tools. Below we explore the challenges of each approach.

Homegrown systems are purpose built by an organization or institution and supported by internal resources. These concentrate on specific organizational aims, specific sources and protocols. Of all the approaches these tools tend to more fully fulfill an organizations' specific requirement at a granular level. Homegrown systems are built for specific purposes, their aim is usually narrower and are less likely to scale to other use cases. Ongoing support can become a challenge as IT budgets and priorities change.

Vendor built systems are purpose built by a third-party vendor with specific guidance and requirements from a customer. These vendors are traditionally service organizations that may offer ongoing support for the solutions built. These organizations often enhance the subject matter expertise available and can provide best practices gathered from internal knowledge bases. Like homegrown systems, service-built tools are narrower in scope and can run into scalability issues.

Productized tools and systems are built by third-party vendors. The aim of products is to provide solutions for a set of use cases validated and vetted by the market. Products provide guidance, training and documentation for users and are supported by the vendor. While products are more likely to scale, they tend to be more generic in nature and may need customization to best fit an organization's goals.

Methods

Processing, analyzing and disseminating data needs to react and evolve at a fast pace in healthcare. Historically, this has not been the case. We are often asking new questions and adding new perspectives to our insight generation plans. Analytical methodology lags, especially in healthcare, as novel, exploratory and discovery methods are a more difficult undertaking when dealing with highly sensitive and protected data. This is a big challenge and a discussion that is not often approached proactively. Traditional methods are becoming obsolete and newer methods (artificial intelligence, machine learning) are still considered exploratory leaving an analytical gap.

The challenge in modernizing methodology is in the balance of continued investment in the analytic methods we use today while creating a culture that is at the leading edge of growth and discovery. Tested methods such as care algorithms (sepsis prevention), resource utilization projections (operating room scheduling), and actionable population care models (diabetic neuropathy screening tests) that we use today will remain at the core of what we do in healthcare analytics. The challenge is in creating discovery feedback loops that help both, healthcare providers and IT, utilize and learn from new approaches. The technology and the expertise necessary to augment traditional analytics with novel methods requires an aligned culture that prioritizes innovation. Discovery processes are rarely tied to direct return on investment and the downstream benefit may be unclear and difficult to articulate and therefore fund.

Human Capital

Successful insight generation needs to be actionable. The deployment of analytics projects and the realization of the downstream benefit requires investing in human capital in IT, SMEs, leadership, etc. and other essential parts of the healthcare universe. The current challenge in this area is related to the landscape of experts available, staff turnover, and the communication gaps between the stakeholders and the technology. As organizational priorities shift so does the constituents of the staff supporting the initiatives. Large and small healthcare organizations struggle to create a balance.

A second challenge is how what is considered an analytics team keeps evolving. The last decade has seen a move towards a more multidisciplinary approach of clinicians, data scientists, statisticians, leadership, etc. While this new paradigm of inclusion is ideal and pivotal in the success, benefit an impact of analytics projects, it often proves difficult to implement and enable as an organization due to competing priorities and communication and process silos.

Opportunities

Tools: Infrastructure, Software and User Interfaces

The ongoing problem with the technology available for healthcare analytics, regardless of type or approach, is the pace of change and meeting expectations. As use cases and needs evolve, tools can become stale. There is a necessary balance between providing insight generation value today and creating a roadmap that addresses trends, mandates and expectations that may be faced in the future. While data collection used to be a bottleneck in decades past, tools have become the rate limiting factor in our capacity for insight generation. The opportunity in tools creation is in the development of nimble and smart systems. Another key opportunity lies in the interplay with other technologies that augment capabilities and allows for a better organizational fit. The pivotal theme is to modernize to a user-centric development methodology that takes into account the stakeholders with checks and balances along the way.

On the other side of the table from the teams developing tools we have the sponsors or customer. There is an overwhelming number of available tools in the market. There are also different approaches to solutions as discussed earlier in this chapter. The opportunity for a customer, internal or external, is to create strong partnerships and feedback loops that help guide and maximize the value of the solution being developed.

Methods

The opportunity in the creation of more efficient insight generating methodology in healthcare is in addressing the analytical gap with traditional vs. novel methods. As new analytical methods emerge there is both a resistance from most and eagerness from a few to implement new analytic advancements. This is a complex undertaking as due to IT budgets, staff and resources, etc. many institutions adopt an all or nothing approach to novel technology, especially around methods. The opportunity lies in the balance and prioritization of goals within an institution and an adequate distribution of resources that leaves room for innovation while safe guarding the tried and true approaches.

The crucial opportunity is in creating a culture that sees the benefit of investing today for the benefit it may bring tomorrow. We have seen technology bring exponential benefit in healthcare. From drug discovery to genomic advancements, healthcare data analytics and research hold the key to saving and improving lives. Prioritizing the downstream potential and creating a supportive culture will define an organization's path towards the future.

Human Capital

To create results that are actionable and create benefit to the patients and the healthcare system, the human capital investment is fundamental. While we may be in the age of Artificial Intelligence, Machine Learning and other self-learning systems, we have seen, as of publishing of this book, the success of these systems is largely dependent on the human capital vetting the data that is ingested and the data that is produced. Technology provides decision support; the decision being taken by the providers and other stakeholders. Healthcare must create, much like the patient-centric approach to care, the user-centric approach to technology.

Defining the unique value of the human capital contribution early in the process of developing analytic platforms and methods will help efficiently prioritize resources and set expectations. Often technology is developed at the expense of the user experience. This is not a successful or efficient approach. The humans involved in the process of care, patient facing or analytics, will remain a vital component of the true value and benefit of these endeavors.

Enhancing healthcare decision making is dependent on the tools available to ingest, process and surface the data. To craft tools that make a true impact, the healthcare stakeholder needs to be part of the development process. Much of the technology used today was developed for other business areas and needs to be adjusted to the complexity of healthcare demands. Technology development needs to include the stakeholder voice earlier in the process and connect along the process to correct as the needs and expectations shifts. Having the right data for the right users, surfaced through the right medium and tools will increase the uptake of technology, the generation of insights and increase the rate of benefit for the healthcare system with the patient at the core.

THE END-PRODUCT: CONNECTING
TO VALUE AND PRIORITIES

The end-product of healthcare analytics is dependent on the data, the tools and the decisions made along the way. Some of the most successful projects in healthcare started with a simple but widely advocated philosophy: start with the end in mind. This philosophy impacts the decisions we make, from the most basic building blocks of data collection to the way the data is presented, disseminated, and the actions taken once the insights are generated. We are at a very exciting point in the maturity of data and tools in that we can ask virtually any questions and will readily find sources and tools to generate insights. Now we are faced with a different set of challenges. Staying focused while leveraging novel an innovative questions and approaches. This chapter explores pivotal decisions and approaches to formulate and answer questions and innovate in the process.

Healthcare institutions, large and small, have different sets of priorities. These differences can be driven by internal and external factors. A healthcare institution's mission and vision are linked to the population served and the impact and footprint the organization sets out to have in the community. While this can shift with changes in mandates and leadership, these are pillars of all the decisions made within an institution. Connecting projects, big and small, to larger priorities is key in creating long term return on investment, value.

Healthcare return on investment (ROI) is a complex measure. Traditionally, other business areas define a financial factor of return that is desired and reported. While some parts of the business of healthcare have a straight forward measure of ROI, most areas require more complex approaches that are better defined as "value." What is the value a certain undertaking brings to the institution? The value can be for patients, providers, community, etc. The term value captures both the tangible and intangibles that allows the specific organization goals' to be front and center as projects progress. Aligning to organizational vision and mission helps to assure that the insight generation creates impact in prioritized areas and populations.

Enhancing healthcare analytics requires connecting to trackable and tangible benefits. One of the biggest challenges is in tracking project progress and defining success. This can be accomplished by proactive and thorough prioritization of projects and initiatives that connect to greater organizational goals. Part of this process is defining specific key indicators of success at a granular level and creating tracking and reporting systems that create accountability. The opportunity for data-driven technology in this area is in creating accountability processes as well as visibility that aligns, connects and realizes and organization's aims.

Enhancing healthcare analytics through data driven methods requires the interplay of many traditional and novel components. While technology will keep changing and innovating in the healthcare world, at the core is the benefit we want to bring through the system to the stakeholders. Creating and expanding on a model that includes the stakeholder perspective as a pivotal part of the process will continue to be the best approach. This will look different for different institutions. Different organizations will have different goals and a different portfolio of what helps them accomplish those goals. What all of healthcare will always have in common is the imperative to maximize and create real benefit and value for those served.

REFERENCE

Executive Summary Data Growth, Business Opportunities, and the IT Imperatives. (2014, April). Retrieved from https://www.emc.com/leadership/digital-universe/2014iview/executive-summary.htm

CHAPTER 7

BUILDING PREDICTIVE MODELS FOR HEALTHCARE

Atefeh (Anna) Farzindar

INTRODUCTION

Predictive models are state-of-the-art in statistical analysis and are powerful for transforming data into actionable insights. Typically, such a model includes a machine learning algorithm that learns certain properties and characteristics from a training set of data in order to make predictions about unseen data. These algorithms often utilize data mining and probability theory to improve their forecasting. Each predictive model is made up of a number of predictors, which are variables that are likely to influence future results. Once data has been collected for relevant predictors, a statistical model is formulated. The model may employ a complex neural network, or just a simple linear equation, mapped out by sophisticated software. The statistical analysis model is validated or revised as more additional data becomes available.

Predictive modeling is useful because it creates the opportunity for insight into future events and outcomes that challenge key assumptions. Such predictors, especially in healthcare, are most useful when their knowledge can be transferred into action. Predictive modeling allows clinicians, financial experts, and administrative staff to receive alerts about potentially dangerous events before they occur,

Transforming Healthcare with Big Data and AI, pages 105–128.
Copyright © 2020 by Information Age Publishing

and therefore help them make more informed choices about how to proceed. The importance of being one step ahead is most clearly seen in the realms of intensive care, surgery, or emergency care, where a patient's life might depend on quick reaction time and a finely-tuned sense of when something is going wrong.

In the following sections, we first briefly discuss machine learning and how it compares to predictive modeling, as well as some predictive methods. Then, we present two application case studies: one regarding the use of predictive modeling in blood management and the second about the use of predictive methods to predict graft futility in liver transplantation.

MACHINE LEARNING

Machine learning is a subfield of computer science and artificial intelligence studying algorithms and statistical models that computer systems use to effectively perform a specific task without using explicit instructions, relying on patterns and inference instead. In other words, it is the study of computer systems which learn from experience.

Machine learning is also distinct from predictive modeling, which is defined as the use of statistical techniques to allow a computer to construct predictive models. Depending on definitional boundaries, predictive modeling is synonymous with, or largely overlapping with, the field of machine learning, as it is more commonly referred to in academic or research and development contexts. In practice, machine learning and predictive modeling are often used interchangeably. Generally, predictive modeling is a subset and an application of machine learning.

APPLICATIONS OF PREDICTIVE MODELING IN HEALTHCARE

The advances in the domain of machine learning in diagnosing disease and in sorting and classifying health data will empower physicians and speed up decision-making in the clinic. The key to improving a machine learning algorithm is solely in the data used to train the algorithm. If the algorithm has a better quantity of high-quality data, it will more effectively be able to make predictions. However, this is a difficult task in healthcare, as data is often difficult to obtain or restricted by patient privacy requirements. Recently, we have seen small steps towards a more data-friendly healthcare environment, including the use of the Internet of Things (IoT) devices like smartwatches to collect health data. This, in turn, leads to major advances in machine learning capabilities, two of which will be discussed in this chapter.

PREDICTION IN THE BLOOD MANAGEMENT SYSTEM

In this application, a Multilayer Perceptron (MLP)-Artificial Neural Network (ANN) predictive model is used to accurately predict anemic status after surgery. The prediction of anemia status assists medical practitioners in preparing the exact number of packed red blood cells for transfusion.

Blood transfusions can be lifesaving and are commonly used in complex surgical cases. The type of blood transfusion needed depends on the situation. Two common types of transfusions are autologous transfusion, where the patient's own blood is collected and re-infused, and allogeneic transfusion, which involves someone collecting and infusing blood of a compatible donor into him/herself. However, allogeneic blood transfusions come with associated risks such as allergic reactions, immunologic reactions, transmission of infections, and increased susceptibility to postoperative infections (Sarode). In addition, the storage and distribution of allogeneic blood products are costly and time consuming for hospital staff.

Reducing unnecessary blood transfusions has been a long-standing goal of the medical community [1]. Reducing the use of unnecessary allogeneic blood transfusions would decrease the complications associated with blood transfusion and benefit patients. In addition, it would reduce the costs of providing medical care [2][3].

Currently, hematologic laboratory values including anemic status in conjunction with clinical symptoms and history are used to determine whether a transfusion is necessary. Machine learning could be used as an auxiliary tool to better inform clinical decision making and reduce unnecessary blood transfusions.

Data: Blood transfusion and blood management data were collected from the electronic medical record of the Keck Medical Center of the University of Southern California (USC) during surgery and anemia perioperatively. This study was approved by USC Institutional Review Board: #HS-16-00504. This was a single center, retrospective study using data on all surgical cases from the USC, Keck Medical Center from August 2014 to October 2016. Data were collected from the electronic medical record of the Keck Medical Center of USC. Intraoperative data were documented by the intraoperative circulating nurse.

The data included seventeen columns including Surgery ID, Surgery Procedure, Start Date and Time, Stop Data and Time, Surgery Specialty, Patient Type, Blood B/M, BM Red Blood Cell, BM Fresh Frozen Plasma, BM Platelets, Results Before Surgery, Results After Surgery, Cell Salvage, Cell Salvage Recovered, Cell Salvage Returned, ANH, and ANH Removed.

Allogeneic blood transfusions included in the data set were packed red blood cells, fresh frozen plasma, and platelets. Allogeneic blood transfusions are transfusions derived from another person. Autologous blood transfusions included in the data set were ANH and cell saver. Autologous blood transfusions are those derived from oneself. Acute normovolemic hemodilution consists of the removal of autologous whole blood prior to the start of the surgical case, maintenance of normovolemia with crystalloids and colloids, and re-infusion of that whole blood when required during surgery or at the completion of surgery. Cell saver consists of the collection of blood from the surgical field, the washing, and resuspension of red cells in isotonic solution, and the re-infusion of the red cells when required during surgery.

Artificial Neural Networks: Due to the high complexity of the dataset as well as the need for the ability to generalize any unexpected inputs/patterns, for this application we used Neural Network and Genetic Algorithm collaboratively in order to model process parameters to achieve better quality.

An ANN is an interconnected group of nodes that simulate the vast network of neurons in a brain. In the medical field, ANNs have been used since the late 1980s, and more recently, widely used in medical research. An artificial neuron is an information-processing unit conceived as a model of biological neurons. Artificial neurons receive signals from input links in an ANN. The transfer function (activation function) defines the output of that artificial neuron given input or set of inputs. The behavior of the ANN depends on both the weights and the transfer function that is specified for the neuron. The cost function (objective function or loss function) is to return a number representing how well the neural network performed to map training examples to correct output. The algorithm's goal is to find a function that has the smallest possible cost.

Backpropagation is a common method used to train ANNs. The algorithm repeats a two-phase cycle, propagation, and weight update until the algorithm gets the optimum solution. The algorithm first runs a "forward pass" to go throughout the network. By using a cost function, an error value is calculated for each of the neurons in the output layer. The error values are then propagated backward from the output, layer by layer until each neuron has an associated error value. The error value and learning rate are used to update weights.

The Multilayer Perceptron (MLP) which utilizes backpropagation training is most commonly implemented in real-life scenarios. Backpropagation networks are networks where signals travel in one direction from an input neuron to an output neuron without returning to their source. A Multilayer Perceptron consists of at least three layers of units: an input layer, at least one hidden layer, and an output layer. The output from the input layer is connected as an input into the hidden layer. Similarly, the output from the hidden layer is connected as an input into the output layer to produce the final output of the ANN [4]. MLP model can be illustrated in Figure 7.1.

Data Preprocessing: In this application, the Data Preprocessing techniques are applied to convert the raw data from the Blood transfusion dataset into a clean dataset. In data preprocessing, we used the following approaches: data cleaning, data integration, transformation, data reduction, and data discretization.

Data Reduction: Data reduction is a reduction in volume with the production of the same or similar analytical results. The following columns were removed from the dataset because they were determined to be unnecessary to the analysis: Surgery Start Date and Time, Stop Date and Time, Blood BM, Cell Salvage, and ANH. Cases with missing pre-operative anemic status or surgical procedure were also removed from the dataset.

Missing Data Imputation: *Models* described ways to impute missing data values [5]. These included analysis of randomness of missing values. The meth-

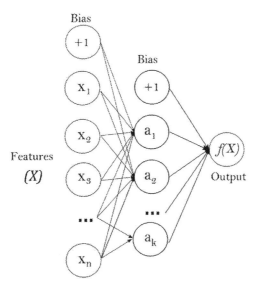

FIGURE 7.1 Multi-Layer Perceptron Model (Supervised Neural Networks)

ods of imputing missing data values described included simply discarding the data itself, using mean imputation, using the last value carried over, using information from related observations, imputation based on logical rules. Our study used mean imputation, data discard and imputation based on logical rules to impute missing data and to clean the data in order to train the neural network model.

Outlier Detection and Removal: Permissive clinically accepted ranges for blood transfusion parameters as well as anemic status values were used to detect outliers. Outliers were removed from the data frame.

Data Transformation: "KDnuggets" explores different methodologies to transform categorical variables into numeric values by using encoding [6]. In the

TABLE 7.1. Statistics of Features and Clinical Valid Ranges

	Min	Max	Units	Clinical Valid Range
Results before surgery	0.00	1403.0	g/dl	3 to 20
Results after surgery	0.00	19.10	g/dl	3 to 20
Red Blood Cells	0.00	72.00	Units	0 to 75
Fresh Frozen Plasma	0.00	820.00	Units	0 to 75
Platelets	0.00	490.00	Units	0 to 75
Cell Salvage Amt Recovered	0.00	71250.00	cc	0 to 25000
Cell Salvage Amt Returned	0.00	9000.00	cc	0 to 10000
ANH Amt Removed	0.00	7000.00	cc	0 to 1500

data, the columns Surgery Specialty, Surgery Procedure, and Patient Type are categorical characters. On data transformation for categorical values, it is suggested that the ordinal method is applied if there are more than 500 classes. Therefore, the ordinal method can be used to change types from 0 to Z values, with Z being the number of unique classes in a given field. In order to achieve a more accurate prediction and a faster convergence rate for building a better model, data scaling is the method needed to apply to the data set before it is used to train the model.

The ranges for postoperative hemoglobin were used to transform values into categorical results that were used as Y classification results. The ranges for postoperative hemoglobin and their classification were as follows: if the value is less than 8, the patient is severely anemic, if the value is between 8 to 10, the patient is anemic, and if the value is greater than 10, the patient is not anemic. Another approach was taken in the experiment. Data were split into two classes that represent "anemic" and "not anemic" instead of splitting into three categorical classes. The ranges for post-operative hemoglobin and their classification became: if the value is greater than 10, the patient is anemic, and if the value is less than 10, the patient is not anemic. The values for boundaries of anemia level are indicated by Keck Medical Center.

Data Sampling: The data sampling method was the last step in data preprocessing progress. Due to the different number of anemic, severely anemic and not anemic patients, data sampling is used to ensure a balance between the patients. By implementing data sampling for larger amount classes, this will increase the precision, recall and F-1 score for classes that have a smaller volume.

Multilayer Perceptron Neural Network Model: Due to the high complexity of the dataset as well as the need for the ability to generalize any unexpected inputs/patterns, we decided to use ANNs. Han and May used Neural Networks and Genetic Algorithms collaboratively to model process parameters to achieve better accuracy [7].

According to the study, the MLP Neural Network is constructed by using MLP for Classification. There are a number of hidden layers, neurons, parameters, input X and output Y used to construct the model. The X value is the whole data set without After Surgery Anemic Results and the Y value is the After Surgery Anemic Results in the data. A Neural Network with one hidden layer can be demonstrated in the diagram below. The features will be X and output will be Y or f (X) in this case. The data can be separated into rows in which the Results After Surgery is a missing value or is not. The rows with a missing value are predicted and the rows with a value present are used to train/test the Neural Network model.

During the training and tuning of the Multi-Layer Perceptron Neural Network predictive model, we have explored combinations for the activation functions as well as a number of hidden layers. The different combinations consist of one hidden layer to six hidden layers, and as the number of hidden layers increases, the accuracy of the model decreases, and the time complexity increases. One hidden layer in the model was not sufficient to achieve better accuracy; therefore, two

TABLE 7.2. Performance Scores Using the Proposed Method (Three Class Classification)

	Precision	Recall	F1
Class 1—Not Anemic	0.75	0.83	0.79
Class 2—Anemic	0.54	0.58	0.56
Class 3—Severely Anemic	0.48	0.20	0.28

hidden layers were used for modeling. In this research, the number of hidden layer neurons was determined by trial and error. Different activation functions have also been tested, which include rectifier linear unit (ReLU), logistic and hyperbolic tangent. The ReLU function achieved the best result among the different activation functions. The optimization technique we implemented was stochastic gradient descent. This optimization was used due to its good result and time performance for the given data set.

Evaluation and Result: For the purpose of evaluation, we used the cross-validation method which is a technique to evaluate predictive models by partitioning the original sample into subsamples of the training set to train the model and a subsample of the test set to evaluate it [8]. In this paper, we used 10-fold cross-validation methods to assess overfitting and ensure accurate modeling. Using 10 folds for cross-validation, the model obtained the mean value achieved performed with 67% accuracy and a 3% standard deviation. Precision and recall performance of the result is shown in Table 7.2.

From observing the result in the approach above, the scores for Class 3—Severely Anemic were not acceptable. The results were unsatisfying because the Class 3 data is only 5% of the dataset. The model did not have enough knowledge to predict for Class 3. Therefore, another approach was used. This approach combines Class 2 and Class 3 data points together to become only one class. This method can ensure a more balanced dataset, and two class classification explains the data set better. The results improved after changing the three classes classification problem into two classes with only anemic and not anemic classes for the data. The precision and recall performance of our result is shown in the table below. The performance of this model using 10 folds for cross-validation and the mean value achieved performed with 77% accuracy and a 2% standard deviation. This model gets 10% improvement compared with 67% accuracy for triple

TABLE 7.3 Performance Scores Using the Proposed Method (Binary Class Classification)

	Precision	Recall	F1
Class 1—Not Anemic	0.74	0.79	0.72
Class 2—Anemic	0.70	0.83	0.81

TABLE 7.4. Performance Scores Using Baseline KNN Method (Binary Class Classification)

	Precision	Recall	F1
Class 1—Not Anemic	0.81	0.81	0.81
Class 2—Anemic	0.54	0.54	0.54

classes model. This model also gets improvement in precision and recall. Thus, there was not enough training data in the Severely Anemic record to train the ANN model for it to predict with good results.

There are trade-offs between precision and recall scores for both classes. Due to the medical application of the proposed model, it is important to address the recall score of Class 2 Anemic prediction as the most important factor for evaluating performance. It is critical to identify and predict the number true positive (anemic) patients and minimize false negatives since it is usually safer to assume patients are anemic than they are not.

The baseline result of the proposed model is by using instance-based learning algorithm K Nearest Neighbors (KNN) with K=1. The performance is shown Table 7.4. By comparing the results for recall score of class 2 anemic prediction, there is a significant rate of improvement using the proposed methodology.

In the application, the goal was to predict the degree of anemia after surgery based on preoperative laboratory values, intraoperative blood management, and characteristics of the surgery. Several steps of data preprocessing techniques in order to prepare the raw data were applied. A Neural Network model was used to predict values in the After Surgery Anemic Status. By using 10-Fold cross-validation method and two-class classification, the accuracy that is obtained is 77%. The result for predicting 3 classes categorical values was unacceptable, due to the small portion of Class 3 in the data set. Therefore, the resulting ANN model did not predict severe anemia after surgery. The baseline is the performance result of the instance-based model KNN with k = 1. By comparing the recall score in Class 2 of ANN and baseline method KNN, it shows significant improvement. Moving forward, we hope to study the learning capability and storage capacity of two hidden layer feedforward networks and to determine the number of neurons required to improve Multilayer Perceptron Neural Network Model performance to get higher accuracy and precision and recall score [9]. With better accuracy and precision-recall, the application model can be implemented to reduce unnecessary blood transfusion in the clinical world. Thus, this application shows how predictive modeling plays a predominant role in some of the major healthcare applications and how it can be used for a greater good in the domain of healthcare.

PREDICTION OF GRAFT FUTILITY IN LIVER TRANSPLANTATION PATIENTS

In this section, we discuss the second application case of predictive modeling in healthcare. This application is used to predict the graft futility and perform survival analysis of the patients who underwent liver transplantation. We first briefly talk about the disease and in the later parts of this section, we discuss how we can use predictive modeling for the same.

Orthotopic liver transplantation (OLT) is currently the last resort for patients with severe liver cirrhosis due to Hepatitis B, Hepatitis C, alcoholism, or hepatocellular carcinoma. During the procedure, the host liver is removed, then replaced with the graft after the anhepatic stage. Currently, organs are procured from deceased patients and can remain in cold ischemia with Viaspan for up to 24 hours before transplantation. A shortage of grafts for small children has resulted in the development of the split liver transplantation technique, which allows one graft to be utilized in two operations. However, complications are common, with rejection occurring in up to 50% of patients. Adult grafts are also in short supply: in terms of market size, approximately 14,000 patients are listed and waiting for an OLT procedure while only 7,000 OLTs are performed annually. About 3,000 patients died or experienced progression of their disease to a point where they were no longer viable candidates while awaiting transplantation in 2015. Since 2002, the MELD (Model for End-Stage Liver Disease) system has been used to prioritize patients waiting for OLT. MELD score indicates increased hepatic dysfunction and mortality risk, with a higher MELD score corresponding to an increased risk of mortality without OLT. Because waitlisted patients are prioritized by MELD score, patients must often wait until they are very sick prior to being considered for liver transplantation. However, higher MELD and more severe liver disease are also associated with inferior post-transplant survival outcomes. Thus, the current prioritization system sometimes leads to the use of precious, scarce organs in recipients that are too sick to tolerate OLT or benefit fully from the donated organ.

Furthermore, transplant surgeons have limited ability to predict which patients will do poorly after OLT because the predictive models available have low positive predictive values for postoperative mortality. Given the uncertainty of the outcome, it is difficult to deny patients lifesaving OLT. Consequently, many physicians rely primarily on a clinical assessment of disease burden and resilience to determine which patients are appropriate OLT candidates.

Deep learning techniques have great potential in predicting graft survival to better allocate donor's livers but there are still many challenges to be tackled. In this application, the Multilayer Perceptron Neural Network was applied to estimate missing values and predict the degree of postoperative anemia status. In 2016, we applied machine learning models to predict graft failure or primary non-function within specific short periods of time after the transplant procedure in order to aid the organ allocation process. The models were tested and used to determine the characteristics that contributed most in the prediction task. We also used a Multilayer Perceptron model to predict the mortality rate of liver transplantation patients up to 3 months after transplantation with good accuracy but poor precision and recall, possibly due to training on imbalanced datasets. In 2017, we studied kidney graft predictive model with a Concordance-index of 0.655, higher than the state-of-the-art traditional Cox model using Efron's method.

The objective of this application was to compare results of the prediction model for survival rate of a patient post liver transplantation for UNOS and SRTR datasets and to develop a prediction model for the survival rate of a patient post liver transplantation to help support the clinical decision on how to best allocate available donor livers to the proper recipients. Various machine learning techniques were tested for effectiveness, with the best models being further developed to comprise the prediction model.

The MELD Score: Since 2002, risk has been measured using the Model for End-Stage Liver Disease (MELD) system. A MELD score is a number between 6 to 40, based on lab tests. A higher MELD score is indicative of increased hepatic dysfunction and mortality risk, in other words, the higher the number, the more urgent patient case is.

Let s = serum bilirubin [mg/dL], i = International Normalized Ratio (INR) of prothrombin time, and c = serum creatinine [mg/dL]. Then the MELD score is calculated with the following formula:

$$MELD = 3.8 \ln(s) + 11.2 \ln(i) + 9.6 \ln(c) + 6.4$$

To produce meaningful and easily understandable results, any measured value less than 1.0 mg/dL is rounded up to 1.0 mg/dL, resulting in a minimum MELD score of 6. While 6 is the minimum score, UNOS dictates that any results higher than 40 simply be set to 40 [10]. Currently, patients with high MELD are prioritized for OLT, but with the improvement in management, immunosuppression, and surgical technique over the past decade, lower MELD patients may derive a greater benefit from OLT than previously estimated. The MELD score at which the predicted post-transplant survival becomes greater than the predicted waitlist survival determines when OLT is beneficial to the patient, traditionally set at 15 based on survival outcomes from 2001–2003 [11]. This risk reduction may mean that OLT can be performed to the benefit of the healthier patient before their liver disease becomes so severe that they may not achieve the same benefits from the organ due to deconditioning and multi-organ failure. Furthermore, MELD does not provide any information regarding morbidity, cost, hospital stay time, or quality of life, and many hospitals still use clinical assessments instead. Thus, while MELD is better than nothing, it is not sufficient alone.

Medical Dataset: In this study, two datasets of United Network for Organ Sharing (UNOS) and Scientific Registry of Transplant Recipients (SRTR) have been used for the prediction of graft futility in liver transplant patients using several machine learning techniques. Later, the obtained results for both datasets were compared.

UNOS Dataset: The data used is collected from United Network for Organ Sharing (UNOS), a tax-exempt, medical, scientific and educational organization which controls the national Organ Procurement and Transplantation Network under an agreement to the Division of Organ Transplantation of the Department of Health and Human Services. The data received is a multi-organ dataset containing data from the US since 1st October 1987. The dataset provided is highly imbalanced, consisting of many more patients whose liver grafts had not failed.

SRTR Dataset: Scientific Registry of Transplant Recipients (SRTR) receives data collected by other organizations, manages and analyzes these data, and supplies data, summary reports, and analyses to the transplant community. Data in the SRTR database are largely collected directly by the Organ Procurement and Transplantation Network (OPTN) from transplant programs, organ procurement organizations (OPOs), and histocompatibility laboratories. Here too the data consisted of multi-organ records from which we extracted the section on liver transplant and received a number of rows containing donor, recipient and transplant information. The dataset provided is evenly distributed and not skewed compared to UNOS dataset.

UNOS to SRTR Feature Mapping: We manually did the feature mapping for SRTR dataset and were able to use the same features which we used earlier for our prediction using UNOS for the fair comparison between results generated by machine learning models. Table 7.5 depicts some of the feature mappings between the datasets. After our pre-processing stage for SRTR data, we were able to infer that the dataset had less feature gaps compared to the UNOS dataset.

Data Preprocessing: We extracted the section on a liver transplant from both the datasets which consisted of records containing donor, recipient and transplant information. Since this study is based on the MELD score introduced in 2002,

TABLE 7.5.   An Excerpt of UNOS to SRTR feature Mapping

Feature name in UNOS Data	Feature name in SRTR Data
END_STAT	REC_PX_STAT
AGE_DON	DON_AGE
ABO	CAN_ABO
ABO_DON	DON_ABO
ALBUMIN_TX	REC_PRETX_ALBUMIN
INIT_AGE	CAN_AGE_AT_LISTING
DON_TY	DON_TY
FINAL_INR	CAN_LAST_INR
DEATH_CIRCUM_DON	DON_DEATH_CIRDUM
AGE	REC_AGE_AT_TX

we consider records only after this year. Also, all patients without MELD scores were excluded in our model training. Research has been focused on transplantation from deceased donors only. We had to remove post-transplant features and other unimportant features decided by feature importance for both datasets by using a Random Forest model which calculates correlated features and scores the features. We extracted the UNOS dataset section on liver transplant consisting of 26,3219 patients with 181 post-transplant features each. We also performed analysis using SRTR dataset including 87,334 patients from the year 2002 to 2018. To handle missing data, we imputed the categorical features by the mode and numerical features by the mean. After the data imputation step, all the rows with more than 20% missing data entries from the analysis have been dropped. To identify inconsistency in the data, categorical values with all possible values from the category have been compared and replaced by null if any of the values were not part of their category set. In the end, all the features containing DateTime datatype are dropped.

Performance Metrics: The performance metrics used for evaluation was an area under the receiving operating characteristic curve (AUROC), F1 score, precision and recall [12]. Each metric has its pros and cons. Only AUROC is independent of the decision threshold (the probability value above which a classifier classifies as positive). However, because certain threshold values will never be used in practice (either too low or high), good True Positive Rate (TPR) or low False Positive Rate (FPR) in those regions will lead to a high AUROC that does not translate to actual good performance. F1-score balances precision and recall and is sensitive to classifier performance on imbalanced data. In certain scenarios where costs of false positive and false negative errors are disproportionately different, the individual precision and recall values are better gauges of model performance.

Machine Learning Models: In the initial work, we developed various models using UNOS dataset, with a reduced 29 features used in [13] to determine which models had the best potential to be further developed. The initial models tested were Multilayer Perceptron (MLP), Random Forest, Support Vector Machine (SVM) and Deep Neural Network. The target variable was binary-valued, with positive instances indicating the graft failed while negative instances indicating the graft was still surviving within 1-year post-transplant. Ten-fold cross-validation was run separately for each dataset to tune the hyper-parameters with AUROC as the scoring metric. In the current work, we experimented on using all available features with our 2 top performing models: Random Forest (AUROC 0.61) and Deep Neural Network (AUROC 0.62). We also widened our tests to include graft failure prediction within 3 months, 6 months and 3 years. Then we elaborated these machine learning models for the effectiveness of prediction include the following models: Random Forest, Deep Neural Networks, MedTrojan and Ensemble Learning.

Random Forest: We developed a Random Forest classifier algorithm using Scikit-learn. Our model has 180 trees, maximum depth of 20, using a sample of 150 features per tree and the minimum number of samples to be a leaf node was taken to be 1. The misclassification penalty for each training instance was weighted inversely proportional to the occurrence ratio of its class to counteract the bias caused by imbalanced data.

Deep Neural Network: We implemented row variants of Deep Neural Networks. The first version was a feedforward network where all 181 features are used. For the second version (MedTrojan), we did feature selection via Random Forest feature importance before passing the input to the model.

Basic Deep Neural Network: Our Deep Neural Network model was implemented in TensorFlow. The model has 6 hidden layers. The number of neurons per layer is all 200. Each hidden layer has dropout applied with the same keep ratio of 0.5. All neurons use the rectified linear activation function. The single output neuron is sigmoid activated to map to probability space. For learning, we used the Adam optimizer [14] with a learning rate of 1e-6. The training was executed in batches of 100 instances for 4000 epochs. Similar to Random Forest, the loss function is also weighted inversely to the class frequency of each instance. Deep Neural Network seems more tolerant of data skewness, achieving much higher F1-score than Random Forest. Despite having lower precision than Random Forest, Deep Neural Network's higher recall led to a better F1-score. There is less disparity between recall and precision values in Deep Neural Network than in Random Forest making Deep Neural Network a more balanced classifier. One interesting observation is Deep Neural Network's improving F1-score when predicting graft failure over a longer time period. Its F1-score increased from 0.22 in 3 months prediction to 0.31 in prediction. One possible reason is that the increase in the number of graft failures over a longer time period makes the training set more balanced.

MedTrojan: We developed MedTrojan by conducting feature selection on the 181 input features on UNOS dataset and the SRTR dataset. The feature selection is done by running Random Forest on the training set to identify features with feature importance higher than or equal to the mean feature importance value. Some important features common to all prediction periods are cold ischemic time, recipient functional status at transplant time, a reason for removing the recipient from waiting list and age of the donor. Only these selected features will be passed to the neural network. After conducting feature selection in MedTrojan, the Deep Neural Network performance improved in all aspects. This observation makes sense because, given the high feature dimensionality of 501 (after one hot encoding) and small training size of 54219, the model overfits. Lowering the number of features reduces the model complexity and serve as a form of regularization. MedTrojan is the best standalone model.

Ensemble Learning: In this application, we tried an ensemble technique which averages predicted class probabilities from Random Forest and Deep Neural Network before thresholding with 0.5 to classify. We also enhanced the ensemble by substituting MedTrojan in place of the basic Deep Neural Network model to give Ens-MedTrojan. The idea of ensembling is to trade off some of the precision of Random Forest for Deep Neural Network's higher recall. The result is a classifier whose precision is neither higher than Random Forest nor lower than Deep Neural Network and recall is neither higher than Deep Neural Network's nor lower than Random Forests. The second ensembles had much better AUROC than all the standalone models with Ens-MedTrojan having the best AUROC. However, the F1- core was somewhere in the middle, better than Random Forest but worse than the Deep Neural Network models. Of note is that the recall and precision were more similar, especially in the ensemble utilizing the basic Deep Neural Network model.

Model Evaluation: Both UNOS and SRTR datasets were split into 4 datasets each, with the same data barring their respective graft status variables. For example, the 3 months SRTR dataset incorporated the graft status at 3 months variable for SRTR data, the 6 months SRTR dataset incorporated the graft status at 6 months variable for SRTR data, etc. Performance varied greatly between the datasets. Random Forest and MedTrojan Ensemble models showed the best results using all the available features for both the datasets. We were able to see the performance improvements of prediction results for SRTR data compared to UNOS dataset which was evident of the two most important facts of less number of missing entries, evenly spaced entries, quality of the dataset and less data skewness. Table 7.6 depicts the results of the Random Forest and MedTrojan Ensemble model after 3 months, 6 months, 1 year and 3 years post-transplantation for the UNOS and SRTR datasets.

Comparison of Machine Learning Models Estimation results on UNOS and SRTR Datasets: Predicting status after three months of short-term post-transplant survival is important as most of the failures happen in this time span. The failure can happen due to some infection as an adverse effect of immunosuppression of the recipient. It can also include the risk of hospitalization and inten-

TABLE 7.6.   Random Forest and MedTrojan Ensemble model (Deep Neural Network) Performance on UNOS Dataset at Different Time Periods Post Transplantation

Time Period	Technique	AUROC	F1 Score	Precision	Recall
3 months	Random Forest	0.68	0.18	0.59	0.10
	Ens-MedTrojan	0.70	0.27	0.21	0.38
6 months	Random Forest	0.69	0.17	0.59	0.10
	Ens-MedTrojan	0.67	0.27	0.39	0.21
1 year	Random Forest	0.67	0.14	0.60	0.08
	Ens-MedTrojan	0.68	0.22	0.50	0.14
3 years	Random Forest	0.67	0.17	0.51	0.11
	Ens-MedTrojan	0.67	0.33	0.41	0.27

sive care measurements after the transplant and that is why estimation of graft status for a short time span of 3 months is very critical.

Table 7.7 shows the comparison of F1 scores and AUROC for both UNOS and SRTR datasets on all our machine learning models for estimation of graft status at three months.

If we consider UNOS dataset, Random Forest's AUROC is slightly better than Deep Neural Network's (by an average of 0.02) but the F1-score is much lower (by an average of 0.12). The extremely low F1-score is due to its small recall values, mostly below 0.1. This suggests Random Forest is very affected by the imbalance inherent in the data (7 times more negative than positive instances on average). The low recall will be an issue for liver allocation in a transplant because a patient might die or his condition might worsen if the classifier wrongly predicts his graft will not fail. In such an application, higher recall is more desirable than precision. This is because they foresee our system as a first cut filter where all grafts predicted to fail will be further accessed by physicians, making a slight increase in false positive ratio acceptable. On the contrary, the same Random Forest and deep neural network model have a better F1-score and AUROC on the SRTR dataset. Clearly, SRTR has a uniform distribution of data, unlike UNOS where the data is skewed. The results (in Figure 7.2) show the graphical comparison of F1-score and AUROC for both SRTR and UNOS datasets on all our machine learning models for the estimation of graft status at three months.

Survival Analysis: Survival analysis is the measure of time to an event. The event can be anything defined by the user and explicitly available in the data. Here, the event they are measuring is time for liver-graft failure. The newly transplanted liver is more susceptible to infections and sometimes can be rejected by the body. Things that determine these are called covariates. Survival analysis handles complications in the data effectively. Things like incomplete data can exist due to subjects dropping out from the clinical trial even before the trial ends, or

TABLE 7.7. Comparison of F1 Score and AUROC for Machine Learning Models for Estimation of Graft Status at Three Months Using UNOS and SRTR Datasets

Technique	Dataset	AUROC	F1 Score
Deep Learning	UNOS	0.70	0.22
	SRTR	0.86	0.53
MedTrojan	UNOS	0.69	0.24
	SRTR	0.90	0.59
Random Forest	UNOS	0.68	0.18
	SRTR	0.96	0.76
Ensemble	UNOS	0.70	0.25
	SRTR	0.95	0.56
Ens-MedTrojan	UNOS	0.70	0.27
	SRTR	0/96	0.69

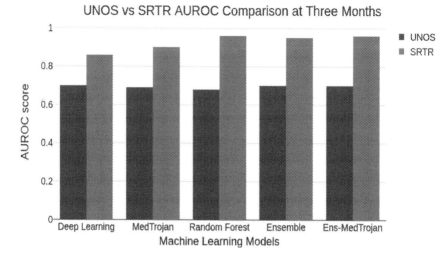

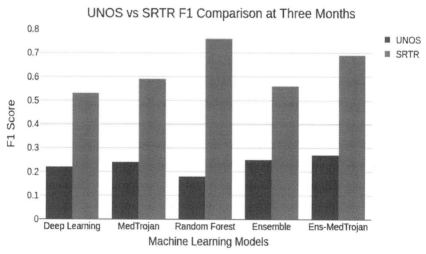

FIGURE 7.2 Graphical Comparison of F1-score and AUROC for Both SRTR and UNOS Datasets at Three-Month Period

the event not happening during the entire course of the trial. This is called censoring. Ignoring these kinds of data would cause generalization bias while testing. The probability of the event happening could be less and that percentage with respect to the entire population under study needs to be captured.

Motivation: After superseding Child-Turcotte-Pugh (calculating the severity of cirrhosis) score, MELD has become the de-facto metric for organ allocation for liver transplantation. MELD has been successful in lowering the importance of waiting time and placing more weight in liver disease severity. MELD score has also been demonstrated to be a good predictor of three-month mortality for patients awaiting liver transplantation. However, since the 3-month mortality values are associated with MELD scores, having a small range, it causes ties to be frequent as seen Patients who fall into the same MELD range with the same blood type would be prioritized by waiting time. We have chosen the range (12—23 for MELD) because the hazard ratio is statistically lower and most transplants occurred during this time period. MELD score at 15 represents a transition point, where the comparative hazard of undergoing transplant versus remaining on the waiting list drops significantly. Beyond 18, substantial and progressively higher survival benefit were shown. It was also shown that since the introduction of MELD in the period February 27, 2002, to February 26, 2003, the average MELD score at the time of transplantation is 24.

From the statistics, it can be seen that there are many times within the 12–23 range. This means waiting time and other factors are still necessary for the allocation of livers. Currently, there are also many special severity conditions that are not reflected by MELD but do justify expedited liver transplants. These are called MELD exceptions and require either manual increments to MELD scores or petitioning.

With this goal in mind, it has been intended to design a multi-task deep learning model for analyzing patient-specific liver graft. This model predicts both the time of graft failure and its rank in the cox partial log-likelihood framework. The model's first output, for ranking patients by survival time, can be used in prioritizing patients that fall in the same operational MELD range. The second output, for estimating graft survival times, can be used to perform survival analysis (i.e., to get the exact time of when the liver might fail) to help surgeons make more informed decisions.

Survival Analysis with Continuous Time: Let T be the failure or censored time. Failure time is if the event happens during the study and censored time is if the event does not happen during the study. The Survival function $S(t)$ can be defined as the probability of an event happening after t.

$$S(t) = \Pr(T \geq t)$$

A more important metric is the Hazard function Lambda(t). Hazard function defines the probability of the event happening at an instant in time, given that the event did not occur before.

$$\lambda(t) = \lim_{dt \to \infty} \frac{\Pr(t \leq T \leq t + dr \mid T \geq t)}{dt}$$

This Hazard value which indicates risk can be used to rank donor-recipient combinations.

Cox Proportional Hazards Model: The standard method for survival analysis before the popularity of Deep Learning was through Cox models. The most well-known among these kinds of models is the Cox Proportional Model which makes the assumption that the rate of risk is constant throughout the study. It estimates the Risk function h(x) in the following way:

$$h(x) = e^{\beta x}$$

where β is the parameter vector and x is the feature vector.

This risk function is optimized by minimizing the Cox partial likelihood loss function:

$$L(\beta) = \prod_{i:E_i=i} \frac{\exp(h(x_i))}{\sum_{j \in R(T_i)} \exp(h(x_j))}$$

where is the event time, E_i is a binary value indicating whether the event happened or not, and is the risk set indicating all the recipients who are still at risk at time t. As the number of data points increases, the possibility of multiple events happening at the same time increases. These are called events. In the below sections we define a modified Cox partial likelihood function, with the approximation of similar to Effron.

Deep Survival Model: In Deep Survival Model, Deep Learning techniques are used directly to learn the hazard function. These models overcome many of the restrictions of cox models like the proportionality assumption. In this applica-

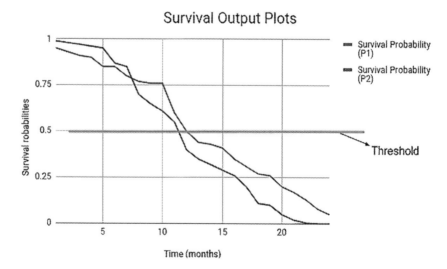

FIGURE 7.3.   Survival Output Probability Values of Two Patients

tion, they analyzed multi-task methods of achieving our desired goal of improving donor-recipient selections for transplantation. Deep Survival Analysis is one of the ways which efficiently captures the timeline of a clinical trial, and helps rank recipients for every donor. Below sections explain details on the model and optimization loss functions used.

Figure 7.3 is a plot of the probability values of two patients, which are the outputs (second outputs) of two donor-recipient inputs. We can clearly say that, after the threshold, survival probability of P1 is higher than that of P2, so P1 is a better candidate over P2. So, our model helps to make these kinds of decisions by predicting the survival timelines.

Model Details: The model was built is a five-layered network with three hidden layers, one input layer and two output layers as shown in figure 7.4 [15]. The model is a multi-task Deep Neural Network with the following as outputs:

Loss Functions: The first loss function is a Cox partial likelihood loss combined with an approximation of Effron to handle ties. The second loss function is a combination of isotonic regression and ranking loss as derived in, modified as in to handle censored data. In statistics, isotonic regression or monotonic regression is the technique of fitting a free-form line to a sequence of observations under the

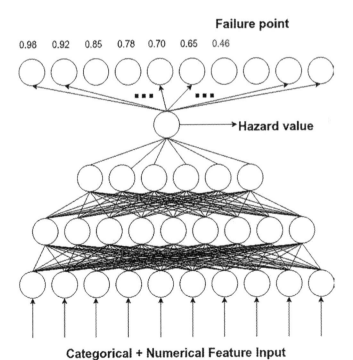

FIGURE 7.4. Deep Neural Network

following constraints: the fitted free-form line has to be non-decreasing (or non-increasing) everywhere, and it has to lie as close to the observations as possible.

The result of the first output layer is just a value, proportional to the Hazard value. We inferred the ranking of patients by comparing their Hazard values. The lesser the Hazard value, the less the risk the patient is in and hence will be positioned lower in the rank. The output of the second layer, on the other hand, identifies meaningful results from the Hazard value and provides timelines of when exactly the event might happen.

Implementation: We ran experiments on USC's High-Performance Computing servers. The computing system has 12GB of Tesla K40 GPU memory. The HPC system has secure servers to hold sensitive medical data, which can be accessed and used only by certified members. Our preprocessing is a separate module which takes about 10 minutes to run and it generates three files—train, validation, and test with 70%, 15% and 15% as the split. The model takes about 4–5 hours to train and the hyperparameters are tuned using the validation set. We use random search to set the hyperparameters.

EVALUATION AND RESULTS

C-Index: For Survival Analysis a metric called C-index (Concordance index) is used. It measures how good the ranking system is by finding the probability of inverted pairs. For example, if are the event times and occurrences in our dataset, C-index starts by counting the number of pairs which are wrongly ordered by the model. C-index is the ratio of this value by the total number of admissible pairs. A pair are considered admissible if is not censored and during the event, itis still under risk.

Results: Table 7.8 contains the results for both UNOS and SRTR datasets. Single loss function corresponds to using just Cox-partial likelihood and double loss function corresponds to using both losses and hence jointly learning likelihood and ranks. The C-index values for survival analysis are acceptable if it is in between 0.6 and 0.7 and excellent above 0.7. C-index of 0.5 is considered.

Intuitively, the double loss function should be more effective than the single loss function since the training is more constrained. The results of the two loss functions should be coherent. It is believed that bad UNOS results are due to missing and inconsistent data. SRTR is a much clearer dataset and we get better results.

In this, we observed that Random Forest has the top performance, with an F1-score of 0.76 and an AUROC of 0.96 for 3 months prediction. It is also noted that Deep Neural Network's performance improves when predicting graft failure over a longer time period. Later, we also tested the effects of an averaging ensemble to integrate the higher recall and F1-score of Deep Neural Network and the good precision of Random Forest. The ensemble utilizing the basic Deep Neural Network and Random Forest models had a higher F1-score of 0.56 while MedTrojan Ensemble model had a higher AUROC of 0.96 for 3 months prediction. This

TABLE 7.8.   C-Index Obtained for the Two Models
Tested on UNOS and SRTR Datasets

Dataset	Method	C-index
UNOS	Single Loss Function	0.62
	Double Loss Function	0.57
SRTR	Single Loss Function	0.76
	Double Loss Function	0.82

system could help on both ends (patient and doctor) wherein the patient can be ensured a longer survival rate and provide a second opinion to the doctor about the amount of risk involved in performing the surgery.

Finally, we presented our study on multi-task learning for developing a deep learning method that directly models the survival analysis function to predict survival times for graft in liver transplant patients. In this research, they compared the results using c-index metrics for two methods: single loss function and double loss function. We used the two datasets, UNOS, and SRTR where the features were mapped. This study on survival analysis results in improved learning efficiency and prediction accuracy for the graft futility in liver transplantation patients when comparing to previous works for training the models separately. The predictive and modeling capabilities of the multi-task survival analysis will enable the medical team to use Deep Neural Networks as a valuable tool in their clinical decisions related to allocating organs.

CONCLUSION

To illustrate the concepts and principles covered at the beginning of the chapter, we introduced two real-life applications in healthcare wherein the first application used Machine Learning for healthcare and the second application used Deep Learning Ensemble methods. So, from these two applications presented above it can be clearly understood how predictive modeling plays a predominant role in the domain of healthcare.

REFERENCES

1.   Carson, J. L., Stanworth, S. J., Roubinian, N., Fergusson, D. A., Triulzi, D., Doree, C., & Hebert, P. C. (2016). Transfusion thresholds and other strategies for guiding allogeneic red blood cell transfusion. *Cochrane database of systematic reviews* (Issue 10. Art. No.: CD002042). DOI: 10.1002/14651858.CD002042. pub4.

2.   Fisahn, C., Schmidt, C., Schroeder, J. E., Vialle, E., Lieberman, I. H., Dettori, J. R., & Schildhauer, T. A. (2018). *Blood transfusion and postoperative infection in spine surgery: A systematic review. Global Spine Journal, 8*(2), 198–207.

3.   Li, S. L., Ye, Y., & Yuan, X. H. (2017). Association between allogeneic or autologous blood transfusion and survival in patients after radical prostatectomy: A sys-

tematic review and meta-analysis. *PloS one, 12*(1), e0171081. doi:10.1371/journal.
pone.0171081

4. Hamdan, H., & Garibaldi, J. (2009). *Modelling survival prediction in medical data.*
The 9th Annual Workshop on Computational Intelligence (UKCI2009), Nottingham,
UK.

5. Gelman, A., & Hill, J. (2006) *Data analysis using regression and multilevel/hierarchical models.* Department of Statistics Columbia University in the City of New York.
Retrieved from: http://www.stat.columbia.edu/~gelman/arm/missing.pdf

6. McGinnis, W. (n.d.). *KDnuggets analytics big data data mining and data science.* Retrieved December 14, 2016, from KDnuggets. Website: http://www.kdnuggets.com/

7. Han, S.-S., & May, G. S. (1997) Using neural network process models to perform
PECVD silicon dioxide recipe synthesis via genetic algorithms. *IEEE Transactions
on Semiconductor Manufacturing, 10*(2), 279–287.

8. Stone, M. (1974). Cross-validatory choice and assessment of statistical predictions. *J.
Royal Stat. Soc., 36*(2), 111–147.

9. Huang, G.-B. (2003). Learning capability and storage capacity of two-hidden-layer
feedforward networks. *IEEE Transactions Neural Network, 14*(2), 274–281.

10. Bambha, K., & Kamath, P. (2013). Model for end-stage liver disease (meld), *UpToDate.* Waltham, MA: UpToDate.

11. Merion, R., Schaubel, D., Dykstra, D., Freeman, R., Port, F., & Wolfe, R. (2005). The
survival benefit of liver transplantation. *American Journal of Transplantation, 5*(2),
307–313.

12. Menon, A., Jiang, X., Vembu, S., Elkan, C., & Ohno-Machado, L. (2012) Predicting accurate probabilities with a ranking loss. *Proceedings of the International Conference on Machine Learning.* International Conference on Machine Learning NIH
Public Access, 2012, (p. 703). Retrieved from: https://www.ncbi.nlm.nih.gov/pmc/
articles/PMC4180410/

13. Raji, C. G., & Chandra, V. (2016). Artificial neural networks in prediction of patient
survival after liver transplantation. *J. Health. Med. Inform, 7*, 1.

14. Kingma, D., & Ba, J. (2015). *Adam: A method for stochastic optimization.* Paper presented at the 3rd International Conference for Learning Representations, San Diego,
CA.

15. Bland, M., & Altman D. (1998). *Survival probabilities (the Kaplan-Meier method),*
BMJ, 317(7172), 1572–1580.

16. Cotler, J. S. (2015). *Liver transplantation: donor selection.* Retrieved from: https://
www.uptodate.com/contents/living-donor-liver-transplantation

17. Collobert, R., & Bengio, S. (2004). *Links between perceptrons, MLPs and SVMs.* Paper presented at the Proc. Intl. Conf. on Machine Learning (ICML). Retrieved from:
https://icml.cc/Conferences/2004/proceedings/papers/291.pdf

18. EDUCBA (Corporate Bridge Consultancy Pvt Ltd). (2019). *Machine learning vs predictive modeling—8 awesome differences.* Retrieved from: https://www.educba.com/
machine-learning-vs-predictive-modelling/

19. Farzindar, A., & Kashi, A. (2019). *Multi-task survival analysis of liver transplantation using deep learning.* Paper presented at Proceedings of the Thirty-second International Florida Artificial Intelligence Research Society Conference, FLAIRS Sarasota,
FL. May 19–22, 2019. AAAI Press. Retrieved from: https://aaai.org/ocs/index.php/
FLAIRS/FLAIRS19/paper/view/18185

20. Fisahn, C., Schmidt, C., Schroeder, J. E., Vialle, E., Lieberman, I. H., Dettori, J. R., & Schildhauer, T. A. (2018). *Blood transfusion and postoperative infection in spine surgery: A systematic review. Global Spine Journal, 8*(2), 198–207.

21. Harrell, Jr., F., Califf, M. R., Pryor, B. D., Lee, L. K., & Rosati, A, R. (1982). *Evaluating the yield of medical tests, JAMA, 247*(18), 2543–2546.

22. Hashemian, A., Beiranvand, B., Rezaei, M., & Reissi, D. (2013). A comparison between Cox regression and parametric methods in analyzing kidney transplant survival *World Appl. Sci. J., 26*(4), 502–7.

23. Jerez-Aragonés, J., Gómez-Ruiz, J., Ramos-Jiménez, G., Muñoz-Pérez, J., & Alba-Conejo, E. (2003). A combined neural network and decision trees model for prognosis of breast cancer relapse *Artificial Intelligence in Medicine, 27*(1), 45–63.

24. Katzman J., Shaham U., Bates J., Cloninger A., Jiang T., & Kluger T. (2018), *DeepSurv: Personalized treatment recommender system using a Cox proportional hazards deep neural network*, Retrieved from: https://doi.org/10.1186/s12874-018-0482-1.

25. Kim, W. R., Lake, J. R., Smith, J. M., Skeans, M. A., Schladt, D. P., Edwards, E. B., Harper, A M., Wainright, J. L., Snyder, J. J., & Israni, A.K. (2017). OPTN/SRTR 2015 annual data report: Liver. *American Journal of Transplantation, 17*, 174–251.

26. Lau, L., Kankanige, Y., Rubinstein, B., Jones, R., Christophe, C., Muralidharan, V., & Bailey, J. (2017). Machine-learning algorithms predict graft failure after liver transplantation. *Transplantation, 101*(4), e125–e132.

27. Luck, M., Sylvain, T., Cardinal, H., Lodi, A., & Bengio, Y. (2017). Deep learning for patient-specific kidney graft survival analysis. Retrieved from: {https://dblp.org/rec/bib/journals/corr/LuckSCLB17.

28. Raschka, S. (2014). *Predictive modeling, supervised machine learning, and pattern classification—The big picture.* Retrieved from: https://sebastianraschka.com/Articles/2014_intro_supervised_learning.html

29. Rosenblatt, F.; (1957). *The perceptron—A perceiving and recognizing automaton* (Technical Report 85-460-1). Buffalo, NY: Cornell Aeronautical Laboratory. Retrieved from: https://blogs.umass.edu/brain-wars/files/2016/03/rosenblatt-1957.pdf

30. Sarode, R. M. (n.d.). *Complications of transfusion.* (The University of Texas Southwestern Medical Center at Dallas) Retrieved from Merck: Manuals Professional Edition. Retrieved from: http://www.merckmanuals.com/professional/hematology-and-oncology/transfusion-medicine/complications-of-transfusion

31. Schlansky, B., Chen, Y., Scott, D. L., Austin, D., & Naugler, W. E. (2014). Waiting time predicts survival after liver transplantation for hepatocellular carcinoma: A cohort study using the united network for organ sharing registry. *Liver Transplantation: Official Publication of the American Association for the Study of Liver Diseases and the International Liver Transplantation Society, 20*(9), 1045–1056.

32. Schlegel, A., Linecker, M., Kron, P., Gyri, G., Oliveira, M.L., Mllhaupt, B., Clavien, P.A., & Dutkowski, P. (2016). Risk assessment in high- and low-meld liver transplantation. *American Journal of Transplantation: Official Journal of the American Society of Transplantation and the American Society of Transplant Surgeons, 17*(4), 1050–1063.

33. Siganos, D. (n.d.). *Why Neural Networks?* Department of Computing Imperial College London. Department of Computing Imperial College London. Retrieved from: https://www.doc.ic.ac.uk/~nd/surprise_96/journal/vol1/ds12/article1.html

34. Vapnik, V. (1995). *The nature of statistical learning theory* (2nd ed.). New York, NY: Springer.
35. Wiesner, R., Edwards, E., Freeman, R., Harper, A., Kim, R., Kamath, P., Kremers, W., Lake, J., Howard, T., & Merio, R. et al. (2003). Model for end-stage liver disease (meld) and allocation of donor livers. *Gastroenterology, 124*(1), 91–96.
36. Ching, H. Y., Bhatnagar, M., Hogen, R., Mao, D.,Farzindar, A., & Dhanireddy, K. (2017). *Anemic status prediction using multi layer perceptron neural network model.* In proceeding of Global Conference on Artificial Intelligence, Miami, Florida, US.
37. Yu, C., Greiner, R., Lin, H., & Baracos, V. (2011). Learning patient-specific cancer survival distributions as a sequence of dependent regressors. *Advances in Neural Information Processing Systems* (pp. 1845–1853). Curran Associates, Inc. Retrieved from: http://papers.nips.cc/paper/4210-learning-patient-specific-cancer-survival-distributions-as-a-sequence-of-dependent-regressors.pdf

CHAPTER 8

A STRUCTURAL APPROACH TO STATISTICAL MACHINE LEARNING FOR BIG DATA IN HEALTHCARE

Alex Liu and Atefeh (Anna) Farzindar

INTRODUCTION

Machine learning is a natural evolution of the intersection of computer science and statistics, but there are many definitions of machine learning. Here, we use a widely-cited definition provided by Professor Tom Mitchell of Carnegie Mellon University. Per Mitchell, "a machine learns with respect to a particular task T, performance metric P, and type of experience E if the system reliably improves its performance P at task T, following experience E" [1].

Statistical machine learning is a subdomain of machine learning heavily influenced by statistical computing and distinguished by the fact that its internal representations are statistical models. Expanding Mitchell's definition, we define statistical machine learning with respect to a particular task T, performance statistical metric P, and type of data analysis experience E wherein the system reliably improves its performance P at task T, following experience E.

Transforming Healthcare with Big Data and AI, pages 129–143.

In the era of big data, the experience E of statistical machine learning has most frequently been to analyze some massive dataset. For most statistical machine learning projects, we do not work with a small set of sampling data, but rather employ special software tools to utilize vast amounts of raw data effectively. Therefore, our focus will be on statistical machine learning with big data.

Statistical machine learning is helping integrate modern technology with healthcare. Payers, providers, and pharmaceutical companies are all seeing applicability in their spaces and taking advantage of machine learning. A few examples of such initiatives include Project InnerEye, a research-based, AI-powered software tool for planning radiotherapy, authored by Microsoft research. Another initiative called Healthcare.ai has developed several statistical machine learning-based healthcare algorithms that provide myriad insights. Google has developed a machine learning algorithm to help identify cancerous tumors on mammograms, and Stanford is using a deep learning algorithm to detect skin cancer.

In the following sections, we will focus on statistical machine learning frameworks, which can be used to compare various kinds of statistical machine learning algorithms and help us understand the technique more deeply. The sections cover:

1. An overview of the statistical machine learning frameworks and approaches;
2. Opportunities and challenges in dealing with big data for statistical machine learning;
3. The various essential tools and the integration of statistical machine learning into an overall big data workflow;
4. Statistical machine learning processes in relation to automation; and
5. A few application cases of statistical learning in healthcare to illuminate some main statistical machine learning concepts and to study how healthcare startups and research groups have employed this game-changing technology.

1. STATISTICAL MACHINE LEARNING
FRAMEWORKS AND APPROACHES

The recent resurging interest in statistical machine learning is mainly due to the same factors which drive big data analytics, including (1) readily available structured and unstructured big data, (2) cheap and accessible computing power, and (3) affordable data storage made possible with the cloud and many other data software systems like Hadoop.

A multitude of methods of machine learning, some of which include supervised learning, unsupervised learning, and reinforcement learning, are applied to significant effect in the digital health field. Almost all of them adopt an iterative computational approach, where a set of computing instructions are repeatedly executed in a sequence for a specified number of times or until a particular condition is met.

The methodologies which drive these computational approaches vary greatly, and it is useful to have a strategy for comparing their effectiveness. Statistical machine learning frameworks solve this issue by providing a unified computational baseline for researchers to experiment with different models.

Among the available machine learning frameworks, the frameworks optimizing the above-mentioned iterative computing and interactive manipulation are considered among the best, because these features facilitate complex predictive model estimation and good researcher-data interaction. At the same time, good machine learning frameworks also need to be supported by computing platforms that cover big data capabilities or fast processing at scale, as well as fault tolerance capabilities. Some platforms even include many built-in statistical machine learning algorithms and statistical tests, which create an efficient workflow for researchers.

To govern how iterative computation gets completed and allow iterative computation to cover all the statistical machine learning completely, a machine learning framework must deal with data preparation, analytical methods, analytical computing, results evaluation, and results utilization. To summarize all the machine learning components and processes, we want to introduce the RM4Es framework (Research Methods Four Elements) [2].

The first *E* is **Equation**: Equations are used to represent the models for our research. The most commonly used term for the equation is the predictive model, which includes regression, decision trees, and Bayesian models. Here, the first E is also concerned with the statistical models driving machine learning.

The second *E* is **Estimation**: Estimation is the link between equations (models) and the data used for our learning. The most commonly used estimators include least squares and maximum likelihood, but specialized statistical machine learning algorithms may require a customized estimator to achieve its full potential.

The third *E* is **Evaluation**: Evaluation needs to be performed to assess the fit between models and the data. The "goodness of fit" metric is commonly used to evaluate models, but there are dozens of metrics available depending on the application.

The fourth *E* **is Explanation/Execution**: Explanation is the link between equations (models) and our machine learning purposes. How we explain our machine learning results often depends on our learning purposes, as well as our specific domain application.

The RM4Es are the key four aspects that distinguish one kind of machine learning method from another. The RM4Es are sufficient to represent a machine learning status at any given moment. Furthermore, using RM4Es can efficiently serve machine learning workflows. Related to what we discussed so far, Equation covers machine learning libraries, Estimation represents how computing is done, Evaluation is about how to tell whether a machine learning is better over another, and, as for iterative computation, whether we should continue or stop. Explanation or execution is also a critical factor in machine learning as our goal is to turn data into insightful results, which can be utilized for massive impact. An effective machine learning framework also needs to deal with data abstraction and data pre-processing at scale, as well as with fast computing, interactive evaluation at scale and speed, easy results interpretation, and deployment.

The RM4Es provide a key method for classification and comparison of different statistical machine learning models. We may compare such models per each of their Es individually, thus reasoning about the effectiveness of different models in a structured and easily measurable way.

2. MACHINE LEARNING WITH BIG DATA: OPPORTUNITIES AND CHALLENGES

As discussed in the previous section, big data is one of the main reasons for the broad adoption and usability of machine learning and its statistical cousin. In other words, to discuss statistical machine learning is almost the same as to discuss statistical machine learning with big data. Here, by big data, we mean data that is big in terms of all the 5 V's, which includes volume, variety, velocity, veracity, and value [3]. Gathering and maintaining large collections of data was a focus when big data started to get attention, but now most attention has been turned to that of extracting useful information from these collections of data. In other words, the fifth V—value—is considered as the most important among the 5 V's of big data.

Big data is readily available everywhere. Per IBM and other research companies, every day, we create 2.5 quintillion bytes of data, so much that 90% of the data currently available in the world has been created in the past two years alone. This data comes from everywhere, with sensors used to gather information, posts to social media sites, purchase transaction records, and cell phone signals to name a few. All this type of collected data is considered as big data, in terms of its size and variety. And now, big data has become one of the most attractive frontiers for innovation, competition, and productivity by most organizations and corporations.

Statistical machine learning is one of the ideal tools for exploiting the opportunities hidden in big data. Big data provides excellent opportunities not only for improving statistical machine learning but also extending the power of machine learning in a way to attack research questions impossible to study in the past, like that about holistic views of customers, as well as to provide real-time feedbacks and interactive analytical features.

Traditionally, machine learning has always been dominated by that of a trial-and-error type of analysis experience, an approach that becomes extremely difficult when datasets are large and heterogeneous. Ironically, the availability of more data usually leads to fewer options in constructing models, because very few tools allow for processing large datasets in a reasonable timeframe, while the situation is changing.

Statistical machine learning can offer intelligent alternatives that overcome some of the problems as mentioned above. At the cutting edge of statistical modeling, fast computation and emerging industrial applications, statistical machine learning allows users to focus on the development of fast and efficient algorithms for real-time processing of data with the goal of delivering accurate outputs. The emphasis now is on real-time and highly scalable predictive analytics out from learning, using fully automated methods that can simplify some of the typical learning tasks. For this reason, statistical machine learning is powerful in creating applications. Big data enables statistical machine learning to process a vast variety of examples, thus building a holistic view of difficult problems, such as product recommendation and customer churn prevention.

Besides the advantages of statistical machine learning, however, there are also myriad challenges for which special tools have been developed. Big data is often incomplete, unstructured, and poorly documented. Despite the recent achievement in statistical machine learning, much more work needs to be done to address many significant challenges posed by big data. There are quite a lot of critical issues of statistical machine learning techniques for big data at least from five different perspectives that include (1) learning for large scale of data, (2) learning for different types of data, (3) learning for high speed of streaming data, (4) learning for uncertain and incomplete data, and (5) learning for extracting valuable information from massive amounts of data.

3. STATISTICAL MACHINE LEARNING TOOLS

To implement statistical machine learning with big data, we need tools that can store big data and tools that can perform learning computation fast. Therefore, in this section, we will cover a few big data storage & computing platforms such as Hadoop and Spark, with which we will not only be able to handle big data and fast computing easily but also build learning systems efficiently, which include some learning systems capable of improving performance rapidly per its experience of interacting with big data. At the same time, we will review a few statistical analytical tools including SPSS and R, as statistical analysis is a central part of statistical machine learning with big data [4].

Hadoop—Hadoop is a system for storing vast amounts of data efficiently, either structured or unstructured. It is an open source tool that is free of charge, but some programming skills are needed to make good use of it. Hadoop is a highly scalable storage platform designed to process extensive data sets across hundreds to thousands of computing nodes that operate in parallel. Specifically, it provides a cost-effective storage solution for large data volumes with no format requirements. MapReduce, the programming paradigm that allows for this massive scalability, is the heart of Hadoop. The term MapReduce refers to two separate and distinct tasks that Hadoop programs perform. Hadoop has two main components—HDFS and YARN.

Apache Spark—Spark is an open-source computing platform, which was built to serve machine learning and data science, to enable machine learning at scale and make machine learning deployment easy. Spark's core innovation on RDDs and data frames enables fast and easy computing, with an extraordinary good fault tolerance feature. Overall, Spark provides two main abstractions for parallel programming: resilient distributed datasets and parallel operations on these datasets (invoked by passing a function to apply on a dataset). Spark is a general computing platform, which contains two programs: a driver program and a worker program. To program, developers need to write a driver program that implements the high-level control flow of their application and launches various operations in parallel. All the worker programs developed will run on cluster nodes or in local threads, and RDDs operate across all workers.

IBM SPSS—SPSS is a widely-used data mining software and has been used by analysts and scientists in many fields since the 1970s. It has a visual interface which allows users to operate statistical and data mining algorithms without programming. IBM SPSS Modeler creates and manages analytical workflows. It was initially named Clementine. Following IBM's 2009 acquisition of SPSS, IBM changed the product name to IBM SPSS Modeler.

R—R is an open-source programming language and software environment initially created for statistical computing and graphics that is supported by the nonprofit R Foundation for Statistical Computing. When working with data analysis in healthcare, R could help make life a lot easier for business intelligence (BI) professionals, including tangible benefits like easy automation, making work easily reproducible, and ease of use with extensive datasets. R's popularity has increased substantially in recent years, mainly due to the rapidly growing data science and machine learning demands. Data Analytics using R is transforming healthcare systems. As an open source tool, R is a GNU package. While R has a command line interface, there are several graphical front-ends and a few integrated development environment (IDE) available, with R Studio as one of the most widely used.

With Apache Spark as one of the most popular systems for big data computing and R as one of the most popular data science and statistical analysis system, there is a lot of effort made to link the two together. Currently, SparkR and SparklyR are among the two most useful packages.

As more demands for machine learning increase, the trend is now going to the direction favoring integrated systems for statistical machine learning, among them, the below two systems are two good examples:

IBM Data Science Experience (now Watson Studio Local)

IBM Data Science Experience is an environment that has everything needed to complete statistical machine learning successfully. It is an interactive, collaborative, cloud-based environment where data scientists can use multiple tools to activate their insights, and easily connect to Apache Spark and Hadoop. Data scientists can use the best of open source tools such as R and Python, tap into some of IBM's unique features, grow their capabilities, and share their successes.

Cloudera Data Science Workbench

Similar to the IBM Data Science Experience, the Cloudera data science workbench is a new self-service environment for data science, which is currently in beta. Based on the company's acquisition of data science startup Sense.io last year, this Cloudera Data Science Workbench allows data scientists to use their favorite open source languages—R, Python, or Scala—and libraries on a secure enterprise platform with native Apache Spark and Apache Hadoop integration, with a purpose to accelerate analytics projects from exploration to production.

In summary, to perform statistical machine learning with big data, special tools are necessary. Fortunately, many new tools are becoming available, and data scientists can look forward to the development of more sophisticated and integrated systems to aid their challenging task of building statistical machine learning systems.

4. STATISTICAL MACHINE LEARNING PROCESSES

In section 1, we discussed methods of comparing and evaluating statistical machine learning, from which we conclude that the best learning systems are always those handling iterative computing very well, or the ones capable of optimizing machine learning processes. To gain a deep understanding of statistical machine learning, we devote this section to statistical machine learning processes. Specifically, in this section, we will illustrate statistical machine learning with some learning process examples in details.

As defined earlier, machine learning is deemed as statistical machine learning if statistical and mathematical representation is used within the model. Some of the most commonly used statistical models are regression models and decision tree models. Under this definition, a statistical machine learning process is the same as the process of building statistical models with big data.

On the other hand, in statistical machine learning practice, no matter which machine learning framework is adopted or what models are used, learning can always be broken into many steps. A collection of these steps becomes a workflow. Essentially, statistical machine learning may be considered as a workflow of data preparation and data analytics steps.

Statistical machine learning workflows can be represented well by the 4Es—Equation, Estimation, Evaluation, and Execution. Before starting 4Es, data preparation is also essential, which involve cleaning data and developing features, while the 4Es process consists in selecting equations or models, estimating models, evaluating models, and then explaining results or executing algorithms, which all can be organized into some step by step workflows with various E elements.

Along with this line of thinking, some people even define machine learning as workflows of turning data into actionable insights, for which some people will add business understanding or problem definition into the workflows as their starting points.

In the traditional data mining field, **Cross-Industry Standard Process for Data Mining (CRISP-DM)** is a widely-accepted workflow standard, which is still widely referred to, even with a lot of existing criticisms. Many standard machine learning workflows are just some form of a revision to the CRISP-DM workflow [5].

As illustrated in Figure 8.1, for any standard CRISP-DM workflow, we need all the following six steps:

1. Business understanding;
2. Data understanding;
3. Data preparation;
4. Modeling;
5. Evaluation; and
6. Deployment

To complete it, some people may add analytical approaches to selection or model selection and explanation of results. The model selection and estimation computation, as contained in Modeling at CRISP-DM, also need to be separated. For complicated statistical machine learning projects, there are branches and feedback loops that make workflows very complex. For example, for some statistical machine learning projects, after we complete model evaluation, we may go back

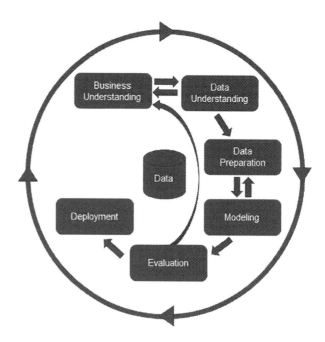

FIGURE 8.1. Cross-Industry Standard Process for Data Mining

to the step of modeling or even data preparation. After the data preparation step, we may branch out for more than two types of modeling with the model ensemble at the end to complete before deployment.

To further understand statistical machine learning workflows, let us review some examples here. In the next section of this chapter, we will work on risk modeling and service demand prediction to further exhibit statistical machine learning for particular industrial applications. For many of these types of statistical machine learning projects, the goal is often to identify causes of certain problems or to build a causally predictive model. Below is one example of this type of workflow as to develop a causal model in detail, with which readers may gain more insights of the steps needed for statistical machine learning or even statistical manual modeling, as in reality statistical manual modeling helps to prepare for building statistical learning systems [6].

Step 1. Check Data Structure to Ensure a Good Understanding of the Data

To complete this step, statistical machine learning professionals often need to answer the below questions:

1. Is the data a cross-sectional data? Is implicit timing incorporated?
2. Are categorical variables used?

Step 2. Check Missing Values

To complete this step, statistical machine learning professionals often need to answer the below questions:

1. Some variables may have unhelpful values such as "N/A" or "don't know"—will we treat them as a special category or throw them away?
2. Some variables may have a lot of missing values—will we fill them in or throw them away?
3. Do we need to recode some variables?

Step 3. Conduct Some Descriptive Studies to Begin Telling Stories (Preparation for Explanation)

Step 4. Select Groups of Independent Variables (Exogenous Variables)

Step 5. Get All Basic Descriptive Statistics: Statistical Machine Learning Professionals Often Need to Calculate the Mean, the Standard Deviation, and the Frequencies for All Variables

Step 6. Measurement

1. Study dimensions of some measurements (EFA exploratory factor analysis is often useful here);
2. May form measurement models.

Step 7. Local Models: Identify Sections Out from the Whole Picture to Explore the Relationship, Using Cross Tabulations, Graphical Plots, and Regression

Step 8. Conduct Partial Correlation Analysis to Help Model Specification

Step 9. Propose Models by Using the Results of (8)

1. Identify the main structures and substructures;
2. Connect measurements with structure models.

Step 10. Initial Fits: Use a Statistical Learning Tool on Hadoop or Spark to Complete this Step

Step 11. Model Modification

1. Use model fit indices to guide this step;
2. Re-analyze partial correlations.

Step 12. Diagnostics by Using:

1. Distribution,
2. Residuals,
3. Curves.

Step 13. The final model estimation may be reached in this step.

Step 14. Explaining the model (causal effects identified and quantified).

The key is to enable the capabilities of working with big data and enabling the capabilities of automating some of the steps to allow constant improvement of the learning, for which the tools described earlier are needed. In addition, it is pivotal to summarize these steps into workflows that are understandable to the stakeholders and implementable by software tools.

Many machine learning tools have features for handling machine learning workflows. As for Apache Spark computing, it has the Spark Pipelines to enable proper handling of machine learning workflows. Spark machine learning represents a machine learning workflow as a pipeline, which consists of a sequence of Pipeline Stages to be run in a specific order [4].

The Pipeline Stages include Spark Transformers, Spark Estimators and Spark Evaluators. Statistical machine learning workflows can be very complicated so that creating and tuning them is a very time-consuming task. The Spark ML Pipeline was designed to make the construction and tuning of ML workflows easy, and especially to represent the following main stages:

1. Loading data;
2. Extracting features;
3. Estimating models;
4. Evaluating models; and
5. Explaining models.

Specifically, with regards to the above tasks, Spark Transformers can be used to extract features; Spark Estimators can be used to train and estimate models; Spark Evaluators can be used to evaluate models.

Technically, in Spark, a Pipeline is specified as a sequence of stages, and each stage is either a Transformer, an Estimator, or an Evaluator. These stages are operated in order, and the input dataset is modified as it passes through each stage. For Transformer stages, the transform method is called on the dataset. For estimator stages, the fit method is called to produce a Transformer (which becomes part of the PipelineModel, or fitted Pipeline), and that Transformer's transform method is called on the dataset.

The specifications given above are all for linear Pipelines. It is possible to create non-linear Pipelines, as long as the data flow graph forms a Directed Acyclic Graph (DAG).

On top of the Spark computing for machine learning pipelines, SPSS and R may be used to improve managing machine learning workflows. SPSS Modeler is based on workflows. R also provides excellent tools to manage workflows.

Besides, notebooks become widely adopted as one of the best systems for managing workflows. With a notebook, either Jupiter or Zeppelin notebooks, computing can be organized as workflows and can be implemented easily.

5. STATISTICAL MACHINE LEARNING APPLICATION

Statistical machine learning is a rapidly developing field. With learning at its core, the field of statistical machine learning also learns and progresses forward rapidly from its own learning, especially by its learning from real-life applications. As pointed out by Professor Mitchell, "one measure of progress in machine learning is its significant real-world applications" [1]. For this reason, to understand statistical machine learning, we must apply it in real-life situations.

Machine learning has a broad spectrum of applications including natural language processing, search engines, medical diagnosis, stock market analysis, DNA sequence classification, speech, and handwriting recognition, object recognition in computer vision, and game-playing. In this section, we plan to discuss two real-life healthcare application cases to illustrate the dynamic nature of healthcare data and demonstrate the challenges in terms of handling complex data, understanding the statistics, and making sense of the results. Then, we will connect these cases with the frameworks, tools, and workflows discussed in previous sections.

In selecting these two cases, a data mining application about identifying individuals with diabetes and the other a probabilistic linkage of healthcare data using Spark-based workflow, we also hope to provide a broad view of the applications statistical machine learning.

Data mining, a combination of statistics, machine learning, and AI has been used intensively and extensively by many organizations. In healthcare, data mining is becoming increasingly popular, if not increasingly essential. Data mining applications can greatly benefit all parties involved in the healthcare industry. For example, data mining helps healthcare insurers detect fraud and abuse, healthcare organizations make customer relationship management decisions, physicians identify effective treatments and best practices, and patients receive better and more affordable healthcare services. The enormous amounts of data generated by healthcare transactions are too complex and voluminous to be processed and analyzed by traditional methods. Data mining provides the methodology to transform these mounds of data into useful information for decision making.

In our first example, HealthOrg (a fictional healthcare organization) is interested in finding out how certain variables are associated with the onset of diabetes [7]. The purpose is to identify high-risk individuals so appropriate messages can be communicated to them.

Applying the statistical learning workflow to this example, we summarize:

Model selection—The decision tree model is an appropriate data mining technique to use for this diabetic data warehouse. Decision trees have the advantage of ease of interpretation and visualization.

Data and feature preparation—Data contains the seven variables of particular interest: gender, age, body mass index (BMI), waist-hip ratio (WHR), smoking status, the number of times a patient exercises per week, and onset of diabetes, which is the target variable, measured by a dichotomous variable indicating whether an individual has tested positive for diabetes. The dataset comprises 262, or 12.78 percent, of positive diabetic cases and 1,778, or 87.22 percent, of negative non-diabetic cases.

Estimation—For the purpose of this illustration (visualization/ interpretation of data), **SPSS** Modeler data mining software is used.

Evaluation—This evaluates the performance of the decision tree model using the confusion matrix. The accuracy rates of the decision tree for non-diabetic cases (both true positive, false positive) are very high with an accuracy reaching above 90%. The accuracy rates for predicting diabetic cases are lower but still can be deemed to be sufficient for this objective. The results show that age is the most important factor associated with the onset of diabetes followed by BMI (Body Mass Index).

Execution—The evaluated model can help identify high-risk individuals so appropriate messages can be sent to them. It can help launch a health promotion campaign to educate people that large BMI and WHR are risk factors associated with the onset of diabetes. This can help scan through its patient databases to identify individuals for further counseling or medical check-ups.

Data mining applications in healthcare have tremendous potential and usefulness. However, the success of healthcare data mining hinges on the availability of clean healthcare data. In this respect, it is critical that the healthcare industry consider how data can be better captured, stored, prepared, and mined. Possible directions include the standardization of clinical vocabulary and the sharing of data across organizations to enhance the benefits of healthcare data mining applications.

Now for the second statistical learning application, it is mainly focused on the Brazilian Public Health System, specifically on supporting the assessment of data quality, pre-processing, and linkage of databases provided by the Ministry of Health and the Ministry of Social Development and Hunger Alleviation. The data marts produced by the linkage are used by statisticians and epidemiologists to assess the effectiveness of conditional cash transfer programs for low-income families concerning some diseases, such as leprosy, tuberculosis, and AIDS.

Healthcare data come from different information systems, disparate databases, and potential applications that need to be combined for diverse purposes, including the aggregation of medical and hospital services, analysis of patients' profile and diseases, assessment of public health policies, monitoring of drug interventions, and so on.

This application presents a four-stage workflow designed to provide the functionalities discusses previously. The first stage (assessment of data quality) is made through **SPSS** [8]:

- The first stage corresponds to the analysis of data quality, aiming to identify, for each database, the attributes more suitable for the probabilistic record linkage process.
- The second (pre-processing) and third (linkage) stages of our workflow are very data-intensive and time-consuming tasks, so we based our implementation in the **Spark** scalable execution engine to produce very accurate results in a short period of time.
- The last stage is dedicated to the evaluation of the data marts produced by our preprocessing and linkage algorithms and is realized by statisticians and epidemiologists. Once approved, they load these data marts into **SPSS** and **Stata** to perform some specific case studies.

The goal is to evaluate the accuracy of the data marts produced by the linkage algorithms, based on data samples from the databases involved. This step is crucial for validating the implementation and providing some feedback for corrections and adjustments in the workflow.

The development of computational infrastructure to support projects focusing on big data from health systems, like the case study discussed here, was motivated by two factors. First, there is the need to provide a tool capable of linking disparate databases with socioeconomic and healthcare data, serving as a basis for decision making processes and assessment of the effectiveness of governmental programs. Second, the availability of modern tools for big data processing and analytics, such as those mentioned in this work, with exciting capabilities to deal with new requirements imposed by the applications. Among the available tools, this application chose Spark due to its in-memory facility, its scalability, and ease of programming.

The workflows in the real example are a lot more complicated, as suggested in our previous section. But, all essential elements of statistical machine learning application have been fully illustrated by the above two examples.

CONCLUSION

Statistical machine learning is defined as a flavor of machine learning distinguished by its internal representation by statistical models.

The major challenges for current statistical machine learning are dealing with big data and making the learning process simple and replicable, for which we reviewed a few tools including Hadoop, Spark, R and SPSS in details in section 3, as these tools make it easy to process big data for statistical machine learning.

Following the discussions in section 1–3, in practice, a statistical learning system is a system built up with learning and data processing tools. The performance of the learning system in making predictions or classifications can be measured by modeling indices like root mean squared error or false negative ratios. The learning system gets continually improved per its experience in analyzing large amounts of data.

This type of statistical machine learning can be represented as iterative workflows, with the elements of 4Es. Statistical machine learning is essentially a process to optimize these workflows.

To illustrate the concepts and principles covered in this chapter, we introduced two real-life applications in healthcare, one about diabetes identification using data mining and the other a Spark-based approach to data processing and probabilistic record linkage of databases to produce very accurate data marts.

REFERENCES

1. Mitchell, T. M. (2006). *The discipline of machine learning*, CMU Report CMU-ML-06-108. Pittsburgh, PA. Retrieved from: http://www.cs.cmu.edu/~tom/pubs/MachineLeanring.pdf
2. Liu, A. (2015). *Structural equation modeling and latent variable approaches*. John Wiley & Sons.

3. Qiu, J., Wu, Q., Ding, G., Xu, Y., & Feng, S., (2016). A survey of machine learning for big data processing. *EURASIP Journal on Advances in Signal Processing.* Retrieved from: https://dblp.org/rec/bib/journals/ejasp/QiuWDXF16

4. Liu, A. (2016). *Apache spark machine learning blueprints.* Packt Publishing.

5. Taylor, J. (n.d.). *Four problems in using CRISP-DM and how to fix them.* Retrieved from https://www.kdnuggets.com/2017/01/four-problems-crisp-dm-fix.html

6. Hastie, T., Tibshirani, R., & Friedman, J. (2009). *The elements of statistical learning: Data Mining, inference, and prediction* (2nd ed., Springer Series in Statistics). Springer.

7. Koh, H. K., & Chye, G. T. (2005). Data mining applications in healthcare. *Journal of the Healthcare Information Management, 19*(2), 64–72.

8. Pita, R., Melo, C. P., Silva, M., Barreto, M., & Rasella, D. (2015). *Spark-based workflow for probabilistic record linkage of healthcare data.* Proceedings of the Workshops of the EDBT/ICDT 2015 Joint Conference. Retrieved from: http://ceur-ws.org/Vol-1330/EDBTICDT-WS2015-complete.pdf

CHAPTER 9

INFORMATIONAL PATHWAYS FROM NATURAL TO ARTIFICIAL SYSTEMS, AND BACK AGAIN

Brian Dolan

We are constantly exchanging data with the systems surrounding us. The most obvious examples are the applications we use in our daily work and our social media accounts. When data is used to make decisions, we promote data to "information," and the notion of information has rich theoretical underpinnings. In this chapter, I will use examples from ecology, robotics and clinical health records to illustrate pathways of information between natural and artificial systems. I will also provide a survey of select AI techniques such as Deep Learning, Genetic Algorithms, and Graph Based Learning to introduce the field of Cybernetics and its applications to artificial intelligence.

By the end of this chapter, readers should have an understanding of system-wide information transfer and be informed consumers of AI products.

CYBERNETICS: A FRAMEWORK FOR UNDERSTANDING INFORMATION

Every winter, chrysanthemums do something fascinating: They bloom. They get up shortly before dawn and prepare their petals for a wonderful feast of sunlight. As an undergraduate helping in a plant lab, I was enthralled. How do plants know

Transforming Healthcare with Big Data and AI, pages 145–170.

it is winter? How do they know it's going to be a short day? How do they know dawn is coming? It was easy to check they weren't keeping tiny journals tucked in the soil, so what was the informational substrate that tipped them off? Chrysanthemums are an example of a short-day plant. They bloom on short days in the winter. What information is available to inform their blooming activity? Given that it is winter, we know the ratio of pre-dawn blue to red light will be significantly different than in summer. No calendar needed. The season has been encoded into the flower and phytochromes can handle the execution [1]. This tickled me to no end. How do systems know what they know? How do I know names and dates? How do bees know where to find pollen? How do genes know when to express? This curiosity is utterly unremarkable amongst scientists. In fact, you could argue it defines what it means to be a scientist. Be curious. Be detailed. Be methodical.

My questions centered on how things learn from themselves, each other and the environment. Shannon explained that messages containing information were being passed between these entities and Wiener developed the framework to examine that process.

Norbert Wiener coined the term Cybernetics in his landmark 1948 book: "Cybernetics, or Communication and Control in the Animal and the Machine." Primarily interested in systems involving feedback, he examined systems as diverse as telecommunications and human psychology. In Chapter IX, he draws a line between a mongoose fighting a cobra to the inevitable rise of deadly self-replicating machines, supported by extreme mathematical precision. He made the act of communication itself a field of intense rigor. Today the term "Cybernetics" is pretty fluid. Over the last seven decades, it has waxed and waned in popularity. As with so much Atomic Age vocabulary, it has been abused and recast by clans of scientists and pseudo-scientists eager to associate themselves with Wiener, Heisenberg, Lovelock/Margulis, Einstein, Buckminster Fuller or other luminaries. In this chapter, we will cling to the original intent of the term and examine how systems transfer information betwixt themselves. In order to communicate with any system, we deem to be an "Artificial Intelligence," we will need to share some sort of informational substrate. Within that substrate, features of the real world are encoded into messages and transferred between belief systems, some of which may be intelligent. Our Cybernetic view will help us understand the ecosystem in which intelligence exists and guide us as we construct artificial entities in our image.

THERE AND BACK AGAIN

We sense things in the real world. We see objects such as flowers, flocks of birds and disease states as existing in an underlying reality that goes mostly uninterpreted. Our brains are performing transformations from our sense to our internal consciousness, but we aren't typically aware or concerned about it. It just happens, and we make decisions post-transformation. I can estimate how far my cup of coffee is from my hand and decide to minimize that distance, largely unaware

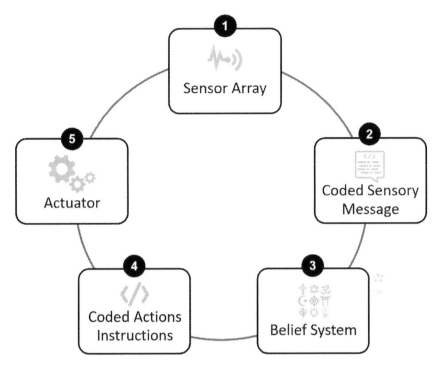

FIGURE 9.1. An information pathway between the "real world" and a single decision-making entity. Here an "actuator" can be any system that changes the state of the real world.

of the multiple electrical signals and binary impulses required to execute that decision.

Let's confront the task. We want to teach computers to make this same kind of decision. We want them to sense, understand, and then act in ways that are unsurprising to us because they mimic our actions. We also need them to surprise us sometimes, or we will not view them as autonomous but as simple Babbage computers doing rote tasks. We wish to train a thing and ask it a question in such a way that a) the query is meaningful to the device and b) the response is informative to us. This means we need several stages of messages from the real world and back again.

To avoid complex philosophy and instead concern ourselves with complex mathematics, let's presuppose the existence of an external "Real World" (RW) that contains perfect information. We are interested in intelligent agents, either natural or artificial, that interact and communicate using the RW as the fundamental mechanism. This could be two human agents having a conversation, a cancer cell producing proteins in response to a therapy or a pig watching a TV. In each case, we have two or more systems making decisions and sending messages to each other. The messages are intended to cause action in the RW to which the other agent will respond.

The notion of "response" predicates the existence of a dimension of time shared by all agents. That is, not everything happens at once. We can relax this assumption, but the majority of cases that interest us implicitly assume a sequential reality. We will demonstrate below why this caveat is important.

Step 1: The pathway begins at the Sensory Array. Typical examples include eyeballs and noses. Less common would be Light Detection and Ranging (LIDAR) sensors, telecom transmissions or neuroreceptors. The sensor array is an interface between RW events and the agent. It is helpful to think of the array as a sort of information membrane. As signals (or data) pass through this membrane, their representation is fundamentally altered.

Step 2: It is crucial to abstract the concept of Message Coding, the process of turning some event into a digital message . We will focus largely on digital representations of data in this chapter, but a non-digital example is in order.

Enzyme accumulation can indicate several kinds of data. In plants, photosynthetic enzymes may be accumulated in response to lighting. Red light, blue light or even intensity can trigger different enzymes. In Pompe disease, glycogen is accumulated because of a defect in lysosomal metabolism. In the first case, "enzyme volume" is a representation of light quality and may be a proxy for time. In the second case, "enzyme volume" represents the state of an adjacent bio-system.

Step 3: The message enters the Belief System. We will not provide a strict definition of this term. It is meant to imply a structure where rules connecting data points are developed and processed. Later we use this as a touch point to define an Artificial Intelligence.

Step 4: The belief system will respond with coded action instructions . Because the coding here is designed to affect the environment, it will reflect different features than the message the belief system received.

The information pathway for a single agent is depicted in Figure 9.1. We borrow the term Actuator from robotics to mean a device or system that a direct effect on the state of RW, like a hand, chemical, image or odor.

The reader will quickly note this chapter holds a strong bias towards clinical information. That is, information concerning patient encounters and the practice of health management. We defend this bias with two points. First, all medical data will eventually intersect with the practice of care. Second, there is a lot of software designed to manage clinical data and thus trillions of messages being sent per day. Clinical data is much more uniform than drug trial data or medical imaging data, making it more amenable to standardized solutions.

SOME BIG QUESTIONS

There are two questions that need to be answered before we can have a serious conversation about Artificial Intelligence and Healthcare Information. These are

(a) What is Artificial Intelligence and (b) What is Information? Let me start with the second.

What is Information?

In 1949, Claude Shannon defined **Information** informally as the resolution of uncertainty. Shannon and Weaver framed it thusly: There is a measurable amount of pre-determined messages that may be sent over a channel. The receiver does not know which message will be sent and the channel may not be reliable. This creates uncertainty in the communication. Once the message is correctly or incorrectly identified, the uncertainty has been resolved.

In this context "measurable" has a specific meaning. To summarize, it means we can distinguish between messages and that the space of all messages is known. For practical purposes, this means finite.

It is a natural response to think the premise of finite messages is flawed. From a purely abstract point of view, this is certainly the case. However, humans have a long history of quantizing the world for the purpose of communication. We have quantized an infinite spectrum of sounds into single vowels, understanding that certain subtleties of pronunciation are of little importance. We have, for instance, quantized multiple pronunciations of the letter "a" to three or four sounds. These reductions are language specific, reinforcing the need for context and expectation in information. Many engineering applications rely only on less than a dozen digits of , which is rather disappointing from a mathematical point of view. In any case, discretization and quantizing are ubiquitous.

And we are forced into this condensation by our use of machines. When we attempt to transfer any knowledge or data, it must be encoded into *features* the artificial intelligence can understand. The condensation forms the *message* that will give rise to the information.

Warren Weaver, in his critique of Shannon's theory, summarized the three levels of communication.

- **LEVEL A** How accurately can the symbols of communication be transmitted?
- **LEVEL B** How precisely do the transmitted symbols convey the desired meaning?
- **LEVEL C** How effectively does the received meaning affect conduct in the desired way?

Weaver goes on to point out that the "symbols" can be letters, musical notes, spoken words or images. Though Level A may seem trifling, it is the crux of many Level B and C problems, and any shortcomings in Level A communication percolate to Level B and C and concludes that this distinction of levels may be specious. This exact same issue confounds us as we develop "artificially intelligent" systems. If we don't consider each level, we are at risk of falling short of our AI goals.

Spoken language is a favorite target for information theorists. How often do you feel you don't have the words to express what you mean? This frustration not only leads to bad teenage poetry, but it also serves as a solid example of information loss from "thought" to "speech." Even languages designed to be technically precise can incur information loss. Medical informatics has generated numerous coding systems like RxNorm to reduce errors in communication.

Medication Reconciliation is the aligning of the current prescription regime with the medications the patient is taking. The medication list is commonly captured within the EHR as a structured field. This field is then mapped to a billing code system like RxNorm [2]. It is straightforward to imagine an automated system in this scenario. The EHR will deliver a message to the system in order to provide information. Suppose the only current medication is listed as "Tylenol, 160 MG daily."

Seemingly straightforward, this example raises questions at each level.

- **LEVEL A** Which RxNorm code should be used for this medication? Do we pick the branded code, e.g. "Tylenol":1738139 (Codes were determined using the RxNav term from the NIH: https://mor.nlm.nih.gov/RxNav) or the generic "Acetaminophen": 315253 as our symbol?
- **LEVEL B** The message needs to augment the RxNorm code with patient information, including duration of the prescription.
- **LEVEL C** An automated reconciliation system needs an expectation of patient medications to associate with the message. For instance, the provider may have a list of allowed medications. If the system doesn't know what the patient should be taking, then the message provides no information.

Our informal definition of information referenced "uncertainty." Shannon was responsible for developing this from the notion of entropy in three flavors: entropy , joint entropy , and conditional entropy .

The **Entropy** of a message source X is

$$H(X) = -\sum_i p(x_i) \log_2 (p(x_i))$$

where is p_i the probability of the ith message of all possible messages in X.

Crucial to the subsequent discussion is that if $p(x_i)$ is 0 or 1, the message has entropy zero and is thus not informative. We immediately know that constant messages contain no information. I like this result because it aligns mathematical and intuitive descriptions of useful: If you tell me exactly what I expect, I have received no information.

The notation has been developed to address messages sent across noisy channels. That is, some engineered system is expecting a transmission from another engineered system. The channel of transmission introduces error, so the recipient has to decide what the originator intended. To that end, the recipient needs to have its own internal belief system that is independent of the belief system of the transmitter.

This point warrants more focus. It is the *recipient* that defines the probabilities $\{p_i\}$, not the transmitter. If I say the word "banana," you may view this as a low probability event and discard it as uninformative, especially if we are having a mature conversation about Artificial Intelligence. However, the previous sentence should force you to re-examine your internal "banana probability" (and that delights me).

As we walk further afield from telecommunications, we need to frame communication as happening between an external source and a receiving belief system $\mathcal{B}$. This $\mathcal{B}$ is the arbiter of information. If the message m is unexpected but at least probable, it resolves non-zero entropy and is news to $\mathcal{B}$.

[binary-info] **Binary Information:** $\mathcal{M}$ represents a coin flip. We are waiting on a message m to tell us the value of that flip. Suppose our model in $\mathcal{B}$ assumes the probability of heads is $p(h) = 0.7$. The entropy of the source is

$$H(\mathcal{M}) = -p(h)\log_2 p(h) - p(t)\log_2 p(t)$$
$$= -0.7\log_2 0.7 - \log_2 0.3$$
$$\approx 0.36 + 0.33$$
$$\approx 0.69$$

Who gets out of paying the bar tab? Before we get the message $m = h$, we are "about 0.69 uncertain."

[uninformative-source] **Uninformative sources** are eliminated by definition. Continuing Example [binary-info] with a two-headed coin.

$$H(\mathcal{M}) = -p(h)\log_2 p(h)$$
$$= 1\log_2 1$$
$$= 0$$

Example [uninformative-source] is to reinforce that a) a constant source contains no uncertainty and thus no information and b) $m = t$ is not a message in $\mathcal{M}$.

What Is Artificial Intelligence?

People have come to view AI as magic and expect it to know things it cannot know. It doesn't. It cannot. We cannot. Try conjuring an image of a two- or four-dimensional universe. Flatland provides a wonderful framework but is hard to imagine. Try it, and you'll find yourself implicitly creating a third dimension in Flatland or removing one in Hyperspace. Our world contains many such unreachable dimensions for any artificial intelligence.

Stew and Sandy have been married for 50 years, are retired and live in the United States. As a gift, one of Sandy's friends subscribed her to a genome evaluation service. The service provided her with statistics on her lineage and other facts about her heritage, then soon began to send her surveys about her health. One such survey began asking questions like "Has your voice become faint?," "Has your hand-writing become smaller or illegible?" To these, she answered "No," "No," ... until she realized: All of these apply to her husband Stew. Her husband has Parkinson's Disease.

Stew had been under observation at a very prestigious medical college for some recent injuries he sustained while falling. His balance had been deteriorating, but the doctors attributed the falls to his age. Sandy suddenly knew better. A diagnosis was quickly sought and obtained, leading him to a treatment schedule.

The institution of marriage was the dimension of communication between a massive genome-mining commercial endeavor and an enormously successful medical college. Thousands of machines on one side, and thousands of skilled physicians and professionals on the other; they linked by a societal tradition as old as civilization itself and almost entirely inaccessible to a non-human intelligence.

So, what is AI? There is no clear definition besides the very dry formalism of Merriam-Webster: "A branch of computer science dealing with the simulation of intelligent behavior in computers" [3]. Likewise, the distinctions between "Machine Learning," "Statistical Learning," "AI," and so on are primarily driven by attribution politics and haven't yet reached stability. This frees us to generate our own working definition, limited in scope to the task of improving health care. Our novel definition is presented below.

An **Artificial Intelligence** is a belief system $\mathcal{B}$ embedded in a computer system. The belief system has the following properties:

- There exists a set of messages Q for which $p_B(q) > 0, \forall q \in Q$. Informally, $\mathcal{B}$ can identify some set of messages as informative.
- Conversely, $\mathcal{B}$ can communicate a set of messages $\mathcal{R}$ that we humans can evaluate as "informative" in RW.
- The feedback system $\delta : Q \to \mathcal{B} \to \mathcal{R}$ has at least one element $s \in \delta$ that is not the identity function and is informative.

Informally, we can send at least one message m to $\mathcal{B}$ and receive r that is neither what we sent it nor a boorish constant. As desired, we get surprised occasionally. It is the last requirement that separates AI from simple information retrieval systems like a relational database described later in the chapter.

In the literature of AI, we speak of training and testing data. The training data is used to build a mathematical model like a neural net or a linear regression. In our language, this is the entropy function H. The testing data is a query q to the model. Does the model correctly respond r to the input? If we told it all cats are black, then ask "q = What color is a cat?" Do we get "r = Black"?

Our definition of Artificial Intelligence separates the intelligent entity from the model being used to execute it and allows us to examine the belief system independently of the implementation.

The message sets Q and $\mathcal{R}$ are fundamentally different, as partially illustrated in this example.

Binary Artificial Intelligence: Consider the entropy function in Example [binary-info]. The underlying model is a Bernoulli Distribution. The probabilities $p(h)$ and $p(t)$ are likely to have been constructed by observing the flip of a coin. The training data may have taken the form X_{train} = HHHHHHHTTT. Once trained, $\mathcal{B}$ is ready to accept queries.

We want to ask $\mathcal{B}$ "What is the expected value of X?" Or, rather, $q = \mathbf{E}(X)$. A well-behaved Bernoulli distribution can provide an expected value, and it is defined as $\mathbf{E}(X) = \Sigma_x x p(x)$ where $x \in X$ and X is the set of all known values. To compute this, we need to encode the values of "heads" and "tails."

$\mathcal{B}$ responds with $r = 0.7$.

Wiener demonstrated in that the mathematical machinery developed by Shannon and others is applicable in a much more general setting. Though apparent to Shannon at the time, it was Wiener who developed the additional layer of mathematical abstraction and called the field "Cybernetics" in 1948. We will rely on his advances throughout the remainder of this chapter.

FEATURE EXTRACTION, CODING, AND MESSAGES

In this section, I attempt to unify the separate notions of Feature Extraction, Coding, and Messages. This is not a general theory but confined to the arena of AI.

Neither Wiener nor Shannon provides a definition of a message. The casual definition is sufficient for most conversations, but here we break with tradition to offer a modicum of structure.

- A **feature** f is a digital representation of an element in a belief system .
- A **coding** c is the transformation of a set of features into a message . Importantly, the coding may introduce noise into the message.
- A **message** m is a collection of features communicated between two belief systems and .
- A **query** q is a message coupled with an operation.

These definitions are compatible with more pedestrian recipients as well. For instance, if the receiving system is a standard relational database.

We may now focus on the practical issues of exchanging information between humans, chemical systems and machines in the pursuit of an Artificial Intelligence.

Feature Extraction

Let's make the above conversation more concrete. Feature Extraction and Feature Selection are central to the modern practice of statistics. Essentially, it is the process of deciding what we want to measure as features in the belief system that is the RW.

California kelp has a delicate balance with its predatory species, *Strongylocentrotus* (sea urchins) and various species of abalone. Researchers at UCLA and The Bay Foundation observed that an over-abundance of urchins prevent both the reproduction and expansion of California Microcystis, leading to so-called "urchin barrens" and unhealthy forests.

The urchin preys on the kelp by eating the hold-fast, which attaches the kelp stalk to the reef. The urchin population should be checked by sea otters, but when the kelp canopy thins, the otters abandon the stand, looking for safer waters. This leaves the urchins unchecked to devour the remainder of the forest.

Additionally, water from lawns and rain interfere with the balance of pH in the Los Angeles bay. Known as "nutrient loading," this creates micro-algal blooms in the water column that make the water murky. The increased opacity of the water inhibits kelp growth. Within normal nutrient limits, the kelp itself keeps the water column at a tolerable opacity.

Researchers have employed urchin purges where volunteers comb the sea floor to remove the urchins. It is useful to study the kelp's reaction to this intervention.

This ecological system, though simplified, provides a model example of a feedback loop complete enough for mathematical examination.

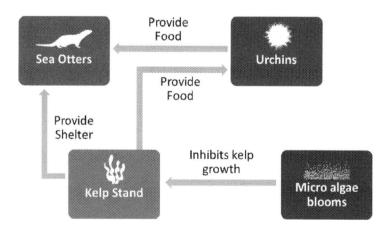

FIGURE 9.2. [ex-kelp-forest] In California kelp forests, otters seek the protection of the canopy and prey on the urchins. The urchins, in turn prey on the kelp. Light quality is affected by micro algae in the water column. See text for details.

During the experimental design of Example [ex-kelp-forest], we need to decide on the set of features. The obvious ones are numbers of sea urchins and stalks. Will this be a longitudinal (over time) study, presumably centered on some intervention like an urchin purge, or will it be conducted across multiple stands at the same time? In the former case, the features "before intervention" and "after intervention" must be present. In the latter, we'll need a study site id or other discriminating feature. If we wish to measure canopy density, we need to record normalization constants as well.

The kelp stand example assures us that Feature Extraction has been with us since the beginning of Science as an endeavor. The perception of trends leads us to us to differentials as features. For instance, the increase or decrease in the value of an asset is an important feature in stock market predictions.

A body of literature exists around the notion of "Feature Engineering," where analysts seek to find insights at the data level towards driving better predictions. The price difference mentioned above is one example of an engineered feature, as is "Banana is the Direct Object of the sentence *The Direct Object has been identified as Banana.*"

When designing an AI, it is critical to identify the kinds of features it can accurately represent. We spend time with this notion later in the chapter.

Coding

Coding is the process of turning features into messages.

Example [binary-info] ignored the issue, but the reader likely surmised the coding $h \to 1$, $t \to 0$. The features are h and t. Other coding systems can be quite opaque.

[indicator-coding] **Indicator Variables** map features to 0 or 1. In Example [binary-info] we saw

$$c(\text{heads}) = 1, \qquad c(\text{tails}) = 0.$$

Experimenters can design yes/no questions and encode the data with indicators. Gender is frequently represented as 1 for "male" and 0 for "female." In that sense, an indicator is a response to the question "Is the subject male?"

[one-hot-coding] **One Hot Encoding** is an extension indicator variable. Traditional statistics employs the notion of *factors*. Factors are used to put observations in bins that have no numeric value. For instance, the "blue" ones or the "control group." These factors are impractical for modern linear-algebra based methods like Neural Networks, which have no ability to understand the notion of "blue." To continue on gender from Example [indicator-coding], we could alter the standard coding to

$$M \to [0,1] \qquad F \to [1,0].$$

To allow for non-binary gender encoding, we add two dimensions to the vector.

$$M \rightarrow [0 \quad 1 \quad 0 \quad 0], \qquad F \rightarrow [1 \quad 0 \quad 0 \quad 0]$$
$$T_{M \rightarrow F} \rightarrow [0 \quad 0 \quad 1 \quad 0], \quad T_{F \rightarrow M} \rightarrow [0 \quad 0 \quad 0 \quad 1]$$

Note that though the gender coding in Example [one-hot-coding] contains the information "from gender" and "to gender," but the vectors do not. The receiving $\mathcal{B}$ will have no knowledge of their fundamental relationship.

[basic-vectorization] **Common Vectorization** Popular methods like Deep Learning and Regression involve data sets that are typically *vectorized*.

- Patient 1 is 49 years old, 223 lb right-handed male
- Patient 2 is 58 years old, 185 lb right-handed female
- Patient 3 is 19 years old, 126 lb right-handed female
- Patient 4 is 27 years old, 141 lb left-handed female

We can encode these patients as vectors by imagining an Excel spreadsheet with the columns **Id, Age, Weight, Is Right Handed, Is Female**. The columns **Id, Age, Weight** are simply the original values. The columns **Is Right Handed** and **Is Female** are indicator variables. Conveniently we can now write this data out as a matrix

$$X = \begin{bmatrix} 1 & 49 & 223 & 1 & 0 \\ 2 & 58 & 185 & 1 & 1 \\ 3 & 19 & 126 & 1 & 1 \\ 4 & 27 & 141 & 0 & 1 \end{bmatrix}$$

Each patient is coded as a vector of integers.

Tile Encoding is similar to one-hot encoding and often used in robotics [4]. The idea is to divide a continuous variable like temperature into discrete buckets that are more meaningful. In many cases, the robot does not need to distinguish the difference between 100.1' and 100.2.' Breaking the distance into eight overlapping buckets

(0,1.2),	(0.8,2.2),	(1.8,5.2),	(4.8,10.2),
(9.8,20.2),	(19.8,50.2),	(49.8,100.2),	(99.8,∞)

to get example coded vectors

$$
\begin{aligned}
c(0.5) &= [1 \ 0 \ 0 \ 0 \ 0 \ 0 \ 0 \ 0], \\
c(1.9) &= [0 \ 1 \ 1 \ 0 \ 0 \ 0 \ 0 \ 0], \\
c(47) &= [0 \ 0 \ 0 \ 0 \ 0 \ 1 \ 0 \ 0], \\
c(\text{horizon}) &= [0 \ 0 \ 0 \ 0 \ 0 \ 0 \ 0 \ 1],
\end{aligned}
$$

FIGURE 9.3.   Tile Coding

The bucketing is not uniformly distributed and is designed to allow the robot to make appropriate decisions.

A DEEP DATA DIVE

We are taking a Cybernetic approach to information and information systems. Serving that view demands we consider all aspects of information, from mathematical models to actual technological implementations. It is all well and good to discuss information as an abstract thing, or Artificial Intelligence as some aspirational idea come to save us, but there are very specific and very concrete measures that need to be taken if we want to improve care or diagnosis through the use of advanced technology. We turn now to some of those topics.

Figure 9.4 illustrates the multiple encodings and messages involved in even the simplest integrated AI. Each arrow represents a message passed between two systems.

Data Platforms

There is an academic subtlety between the terms **Data Platform** and **Information Retrieval System** that will we ignore. The latter is a misnomer anyway in

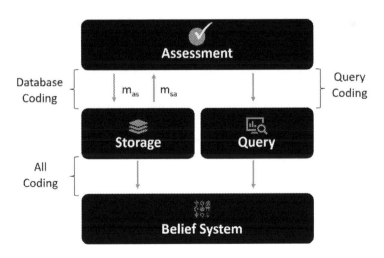

FIGURE 9.4.   Data Lifecycle

light of the strict definition of Information. Each platform has nuances to how and what data can be stored within it.

The Electronic Health Record typically captures data in a data warehouse. Traditionally this means a large Relational Database Management System (RDBMS). RDBMS have been around for decades and are battle-hardened for the task. However, the culture of data management was designed around specific business needs under a very different technological environment.

Storage space—the number of Gigabytes the system has available—has been a key concern for data warehouses until recently. That lead to painful conversations about which data gets kept and which discarded. In the clinical setting, this meant preserving billing-oriented data in favor of patient health and wellness data. In research settings, it meant older data was discarded to make room for newer studies.

As data storage becomes cheaper, more data will be preserved. This does not necessarily mean it will ever become information. Anyone attempting to learn from this data will need to be involved in the indexing strategy.

The most commercially successful data platforms are Relational Database Management Systems (RDBMS). Examples include Oracle, SQL Server, MySQL, PostgreSQL, and Teradata. Each of these provides an interface to the underlying data via a programming language called "Structured Query Language" (SQL). Internally, an RDBMS stores the data in large tables and creates links (relationships) between these tables called foreign keys. These systems have been driving business applications since the 1980s and can be quite powerful.

From an information point of view, RDBMS requires an *a priori* schema for each table. They cannot be surprised by data, and they can never say "I don't know" when queried (This is an essential aspect of ACID requirements).

To add additional data to an RDBMS, the user must know the pre-determined schema and how the new data relates to the existing data in an unambiguous way. This discipline is crucial to maintaining a database of record. A new clinical record will be divided into multiple tables storing the patient personal details, the medications ordered, time and place of encounter, etc., all in separate tables.

A typical query involves asking for all records meeting a criterion like "provider name" and getting large sheets of structured data in response.

The schema restriction of RDBMS leads to the "No-SQL" movement in the early 2000s. Examples include Hadoop, MongoDB, Redis, and HBase. These platforms permitted the insertion of almost any digital medium but sacrificed strict ACID compliance. Also, data relationships are much more loosely managed and can lead quickly to information loss.

Since the input data is not divided into constituents as in an RDBMS, a query usually returns the entire record in the same format it was input. Though summary statistics such as volumes and counts are easy to obtain, it is very difficult to get the linkages between records in these systems.

Graph databases like Neo4J provide an intermediary between strictly regulated schemas of RDBMS and their NoSQL cousins. They focus on storing data as nodes (or vertices) and creating edges between them. The edges are distinct from RDBMS foreign keys in that they exist between two data points, not between two tables. A notable strength of graph systems is their ability to traverse networks very quickly, which are valuable for queries such as finding shared connections between two symptoms.

Entering data into a graph database occurs at two levels. Generally, the nodes are entered first, then the links between the nodes are entered. This flexibility has the advantage that any one node or object and have an arbitrary set of connections. The disadvantage comes from understanding what kind of links exists during the analytic process. Queries typically return single objects that are linked to a certain desired property.

Finally, search engines such as ElasticSearch and Solr / Lucene have gained prominence in recent years. Full-text search (FTS) is a powerful way to interact with data and is the expected experience with systems like Google. It is only recently being introduced in a clinical setting. Data insertion is simply adding the full text of the record. Retrieval is often done by matching words or phrases that stand out as unusual.

FTS has opened the door to very advanced Natural Language Processing (NLP) methods for examining data. As NLP continues to understand the medical realm, it will become a valuable part of all AI systems.

The variety of platforms induces a variety of message families. Sophisticated AI systems draw on multiple platforms to provide them the correct data. However, it is a daunting task for an institution to manage multiple platforms. In this way, the chosen data platform becomes a crucial part of the Cybernetic view. It is the garden in which the AI grows and must be tendered with care.

The Health of Stored Health Records

Electronic Health Records. Most hospitals and providers systems in the United States have been incentivized to migrate their record keeping systems to an electronic format. Current commercial examples include Epic and Cerner, though the fields are rapidly expanding.

The incentives were based largely around billing, so it is no surprise that the systems are keenly adapted to assist in the billing department. Many physicians will rapidly agree that in clinical data, representing the actual health of the patient, is routinely downplayed in these systems. For almost a decade, industry analysts have attributed physician burn-out to the tremendous amount of electronic paperwork that has been heaped upon clinicians. Additionally, patient satisfaction has been reduced because doctors are forced to pay attention to data entry during consultations instead of the patient in the room.

This mismatch of priorities has two important manifestations. First, there is no structured field for the overall health of the patient. If the patient is feeling "fatigued" to "just crappy all the time," the physician has no standard way to enter it. She ends up typing the same note she would have written by hand a few years earlier, except the note is now harder to retrieve than an ordinary paper file.

Second, a great deal of emphasis is placed on the fields that pertain to billing, including medications, tests, and scheduling. This load conscripts the time that may have been spent thinking about the state of the patient, so less actual examination is being performed. There is no standard way of capturing "outcomes" for a patient. This is partially due to there being no real financial incentive to monitor outcomes as of 2018.

The physician ends the exam learning less about the patient. Despite the incredible volume of medical data being generated each day, it is not clear if we are capturing more information.

This data is harvested and stored. In 2012, a study was performed on enterprise data that concluded that fewer than 1% of stored data is ever analyzed [5]. If medical data follows this same pattern, then 99% of data collection and EHR effort is wasted and will never serve to improve patient care.

When we start talking about Artificial Intelligence in health care, we need to appreciate that 99% of the data is essentially worthless. Can we make it valuable with more sophisticated technology? If we are failing to track the efficacy of treatments at the patient level, we have little reason to hope any technology will save us.

The clinical systems are designed to collect the wrong features, the care providers are not incentivized to accurately record patient health, and the methods we discuss below typically require us to degrade the information before the analysis even begins. But all is not lost.

Fast Healthcare Interoperability Resources

A significant problem with EHR is that they are collected into their own local databases, so data is kept just at the hospital or at the provider level. A patient may be seeing multiple providers all with different provider records.

FHIR stands for "Fast Healthcare Interoperability Resources" and is typically spoken to sound like "fire." To the layperson, it is a message template for exchanging medical records. An FHIR message has mandatory fields. It enjoys strong support at the Federal level in the United States and aspires to provide universal data exchange between all health record systems. Standard message templates make it easy to transfer data from one system to another. It is hoped that, once adopted, FHIR will make the sharing of patient data instantaneous and mostly painless.

AI METHODS: WHAT THEY CAN AND CANNOT ENCODE

In terms of modeling, care must be taken to match the mathematical model with the character of the data. This is challenging considering the diversity of fauna in sea of artificial intelligence. It is okay to not trust the computer. It is okay to not trust the researcher who tells you his algorithm will solve your problem. Though

AI can be tremendously effective in many domains, is it effective in yours? The following anecdote illustrates a key problem with all Artificial Intelligence solutions.

[sharief] **Clinical Diagnosis** On of the challenges with the application of AI in medicine is making sure that the data is available to the AI to use. The majority of the information contained in the medical record is recorded in non-discrete elements, i.e., free text. Another challenge is when vital information is never recorded in the medical record. An example of this was a case of an infant with weakness that we were evaluating, but the diagnosis was evading the team. Several times, the father had been at bedside when the child was seen, and it was not until we happened to meet the mother, that I noted that her speech was hypernasal (nasally pitched) and hypophonic (soft) and that when I shook her hand she had myotonia (difficulty releasing her grip). These features which had been observed by the general pediatrician, but they did not have the specialist expertise to identify them as being pathological and to record in the medical record. Once the neurology team discovered these maternal features, it was clear, the most likely diagnosis myotonic dystrophy for the patient and that the mother was also affected.

To Dr. Sharief Taraman, MD, who is a Pediatric Neurologist and Medical Informaticist, the solution presented itself in an "a-ha!" moment. In the pursuit of the diagnosis of the infant, he was able to tap into a complex web of information based on his training and personal experience. For a non-human intelligence to reach this same conclusion would require a very specific kind of encoding.

At the disease level, the AI needs to understand the triple of symptoms, hypernasal speech, hypophonic speech, and myotonia, are indicators of myotonic dystrophy.

At the patient level, the AI needs the ability to connect general weakness with the notion of myotonia. Considering the patient is an infant, this may be very difficult to do.

At the environmental level, the AI needs to understand two critical factors. First, there is another entity that exhibits all the symptoms of myotonic dystrophy. Second, the state of that second entity may affect the state of the patient.

At the data level, all discrete notions mentioned above to be recorded as manipulable objects. In AI, this means there has to be an element of the feature space for "hypernasal speech" to "one entity's effect on another." This is no mean feat.

At the cybernetic (systems information) level, the AI needs to appreciate the interplay of disease, patient and environmental systems.

Logistic Regression and Support Vector Machines

Logistic Regression (LR) has powered decades of simple binary decisions and has been one of the most popular methods since it was proposed in the 1950s [6]. LR is frequently used as the final layer in many variants of Deep Learning techniques, and its popularity is driven by a number of conveniences.

First, the entire method can be reduced to a series of matrix transformations, and that means it has a lot of mathematical machinery to support it. Second, data is often collected as a series of columns per observation, and this is exactly how matrix-based methods like it. It doesn't require much messaging of the data to apply any regression or SVM. For instance, LR is able to directly ingest the coding of Example [basic-vectorization].

Given a data set X and a set of observations $y \in \{0,1\}$, both LR and SVMs provide a probability p that a new data point will have observation 0 or 1. Coding must exist between the two desired states and $\{0,1\}$.

To apply LR to Example [sharief], we could create indicator vectors for **Hypernasal Speech, Hypophonic Speech, Myotonia** for the state of the patient and map **Afflicted** $\rightarrow 1$, **Unafflicted** $\rightarrow 0$. We would have a highly specific linear classifier.

In practice, it's common to have large ensembles of linear classifiers each finely tuned to a single issue, like the presence of a specific disease. The resulting $\mathcal{B}$ is expecting a rather small message space. The queries you can give it are also very limited, mostly just asking for a prediction of a given state vector.

Artificial Neural Networks

Artificial Neural Nets (ANN) are attractive because they mimic the way we believe the brain works. The interest in artificial neural networks may stem from how similar they are to our rather slender understanding of natural neural networks. Of course, natural NN have experienced millions of years of refinement through the natural selection process whereas ANNs are unlikely to reach this kind of maturity. Still, the similarities are fairly encouraging and a testament to our current state of science. ANN were inspired by the Perceptron, which was developed in the 1950s at the Office of Naval Research [7].

Proponents of neural networks will be quick to point out that they are a biologically inspired and imminently flexible form of AI. Figure 9.5 is a typical visualization of a neural network. This network has three layers. From left to right, they are the "input," "hidden," and "output" layers. Practitioners speak of the topology of the network and the number of neurons (circles) in each layer (vertical column) along with the connectivity scheme. In this diagram, the solid figures are activated and propagate signals forward to the output layer and lines indicates which neurons can communicate.

Harkening back to our discussion of coding, the input message is a binary vector. A 1 activates the neuron, so this diagram is illustrating $m = [1 \ 1 \ 0 \ 1 \ 0 \ 0 \ 0]$ and $r = [1 \ 1 \ 0 \ 1]$. The coding almost certainly different for the input and output layers. NN are particularly good at classification tasks, so this figure may represent an arbitrary 7-dimensional vector being classified into three different classes.

It is not mathematically impossible to incorporate values other than 0 and 1 into the input vectors. It does create some mathematical problems downstream, however. For this reason, the features presented to a NN tend to be flat. e.g., they don't hierarchical or relational data like "patient is the daughter of the second

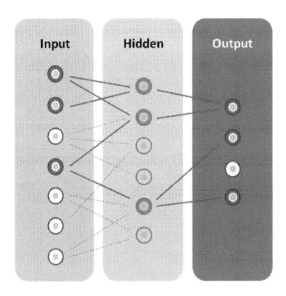

FIGURE 9.5.   A Typical Visualization of Neural Network

entity." This is not unique to neural nets but coupled with the binary encodings it limits the structure of the analysis.

Please note from the figure that any one input neuron can participate in the firing of multiple hidden layer neurons. As the training progresses, the connections are re-weighted to fit the data. In this way, neural nets can capture co-linearities within the data. The training does not guarantee the connections will have physical meaning; however, they are simply artifacts of the optimization algorithm.

At the moment, a piece of data is passed into a neural net, and much of the underlying information is lost. In fact, information is often lost before it is digitized. A physician may record a dosage of aspirin and a test for blood pressure, but never note these two data points are related to a single condition. It is left for the AI to reconstruct the relationship between the two. In some cases, this is easily accomplished, but oftentimes it is impossible.

Likewise, extracting information from the model can be challenging. If the machine didn't know about the correlations on the way in, it is unlikely to know them on the way out. For Example, [sharief], coding the mother-daughter relationship would be intractable over more than a few entities. One would have to reduce the vector to an indicator for "mother has myotonic dystrophy," which makes the exercise tautological.

Deep Learning

Deep Learning re-emerged as a powerful technique in 2009 when Hinton and others were able to use advances in Graphical Processing Units (GPUs) to train the network at tremendous speeds [8]. The method had been developed in the

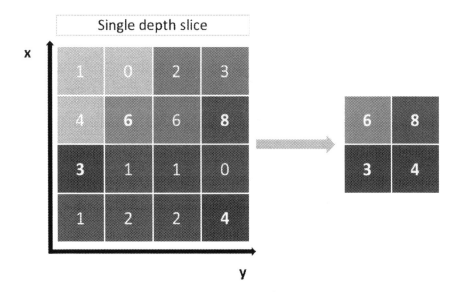

FIGURE 9.6.   An Example of the "Convolutional" Part of Convolution Neural Net

1980s, but the required computation had prevented it from reaching a wide audience.

Briefly, Deep Learning involves the use of multiple layers of ANNs coupled with a final discriminated layer like Logistic Regression. Deep Learning results are as extraordinary as their complexity, and this innovation has transformed the field of image processing.

As ensembles of ANNs, they are subject to the same informational restraints, but this method tolerates non-binary vectors. It is worth the diversion to examine how the coding is performed for image processing as it is a) quite clever, and b) an interesting study of derived features.

A Convolutional Neural Net (CNN) is a member of the ANN family. The "convolutional" part is the summarization of local data. A digital image can be viewed as a matrix of RGB intensities. In Figure 9.6, we see that each quadrant of the left matrix is reduced to its maximum value to produce the right matrix. These convolved values are presented to the Deep Learning pipeline as $m = [6\ 8\ 3\ 4]$ In our current verbiage, the vector has been derived from the source image during the coding process.

This method will not capture hierarchical data, but that is not necessary for image classification. It can detect very nuanced features like ragged cell walls and classify the image accordingly. Thus, a query to a trained CNN would send the pixel values of an image and receive a classification vector.

Time Series

Time Series analysis is another mathematically rich field of AI. It enjoys a number of benefits many of the contemporary techniques envy. First, there is a substantial body of addressable problems, the stock market being just a small fraction of these. The large number of problems brings a large amount of training data, so they know when they get it right and can continuously refine the techniques.

The more popular time series techniques are based on regression, so the mathematical underpinnings are comprehensive. One family, in particular, is the ARIMA models which focus on a few unique features.

- **Auto-Regressive** (AR) is the direct influence of yesterday's value on today's value.
- **Integrated** (I) values are the lag values to account for periodicity in the data. For instance, the values "every Sunday" and each periodic element is given its own feature.
- **Moving Average** (MA) is the average of the recent history of the series as an independent feature.

The ARIMA feature space includes all recorded values for the series with an indexing dimension of time to enforce provenance. Thus, for relatively simple coding of the training data, one receives a beautiful diaspora of responses.

This list is not exhaustive. The commercial impact of time series is so tremendous that entire careers can be spent developing within a single family. Consider that all electronic communication, and indeed Shannon and Weiner's original works, are based on electronic communication and Fourier Series. Fourier Series allowed engineers to encode rather ephemeral features like light, sound and even action into mathematical structures. This opened up whole universes of sensor data to investigation by natural and artificial intelligences.

Time series analysis can also provide some unique and very complicated responses to queries. Not only does the method allow for predicting tomorrow's value, but one can predict a confidence interval around that value, leading to fan charts of likely futures. This is a level of analytic power very few methods can boast. It's hard to over-state how mathematically interesting these studies can be.

Genetic Algorithms

Biology has inspired us to think that the right strategy is out there, somewhere, if we can just figure it out. Evolutionary pressure has brought us to many arbitrary but useful conclusions. Two legs are a good form of locomotion. Oxygen can be used to store energy. Eating other organisms saves you time obtaining resources. All of this depends on identifying the right survival strategy. But the number of strategies is not only beyond comprehension, but it is also beyond our ability to compute. If we wish to teach a machine how to behave in a complex environment, we need to examine billions of potential strategies.

Genetic Algorithms (GA) are a family of AI models designed to exploit the notion of competitive games. At a high level, it's very simple. Start with a large population of creatures (or agents) with genotypes and see who wins. The winners get to procreate to the next epoch. Proceed with the bloodbath until some form of stability is achieved and call that your strategy. GA is famous for delightfully surprising solutions to complex problems. The "evolved antenna" is perhaps the best-known example. The shape of the antenna was developed by postulating shapes and modeling receptive capabilities over hundreds of billions of options.

Traditional Game Theory has provided us with theoretical frameworks for evaluating a strategy. In the 1970s, Game Theory developed a biological nature in the form of "Evolutionary Game Theory." The focus turned from closed games, for which "Nash Equilibrium" was developed, to contests amongst members of a population. An important feature of Evolutionary Games is that the strategy obeys no master beyond "fitness." e.g., it does not have to make sense in any other form. It may not be rational, it may not be optimal, and it may not be persistent, it only needs to be the winner of the current epoch.

When evaluating strategies determined by GA, there are some crucial questions to ask. What is the fitness function? What is the available genetic space? How is the crossover (the sharing of genotypes by two or more parents) determined? How is the mutation (the imperfect replication of the parent genotype)

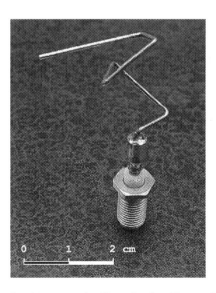

FIGURE 9.7. The Evolved Antenna. Its Charming but Bizarre Shape Was Developed Through an Artificial Form of Natural Selection

handled? These, along with the programmatically technical issues, inform the artistry of building GA.

For an AI consumer, GA products can be quite challenging. The key consideration is whether you agree with the definition of fitness. Was the game set up to create the correct pressures on the genotype? If your goal is high radio receptivity, then the evolved antenna solves your problem. You will never know, however, if it is the optimal solution, only that it works very well, and it beats everything else the computer can think of.

GA as a field is very complex, and the reader is advised to spend some time with John Hollands' "Adaptation in Natural and Artificial Systems" [9]—an extremely thought-provoking and ground-breaking work.

Graph Based Learning

Most analytic innovations experience slow adoption due to gaps in the technology stack. Graph Based Learning (GBL) is no exception. Current technology has difficulty managing very large graph structures across multiple node and machine. It is difficult to predict which nodes will need to communicate and thus which servers need to host which subsets of the data. Recent advances in High-Performance Computing may turn the tide in favor of GBL.

When we speak of graphs in this context, we mean a network of nodes connected by edges (This distinction is important to de-couple from the graph-based execution flows of Tensorflow and other packages.). Graph analytics are distinct from graph databases. A graph database stores data in a format that makes relationships first-class objects. Graph analytics are mathematical techniques designed to find patterns within network data.

Decision Trees are a well-known example of Directed (edges go one way) Acyclic (the edges don't point back to parents) Graphs, or DAGs. See Figure 9.8 as an example. In a Decision Tree, each node represents a single decision, and the outbound edges lead to new choices. Typically, these trees are inferred from data and not provided as graphs.

Like Time Series, Graphs bring about a set of unique features. Nodes within a graph have a notion of betweenness that illustrates how often this node lies on the path between other nodes. For instance, do food webs pass through urchins on their way to kelp? The diameter of the graph is the longest path between two nodes, and connectedness tells us how isolated a subgraph may be.

PageRank is probably the best-known graph analytic, being the mathematical machinery underlying Google search algorithms. Another significant analytic is called **Community Detection**. A community is a subset of the nodes of a graph that is more strongly connected to each other than to the rest of the graph, like the clustering of disease symptoms. For a larger treatment of Community Detection, see Kolaczyk [10].

Graphs can capture an enormous variety of features with a transparent encoding. With a graph, we can finally encode Example [ex-kelp-forest] and Example

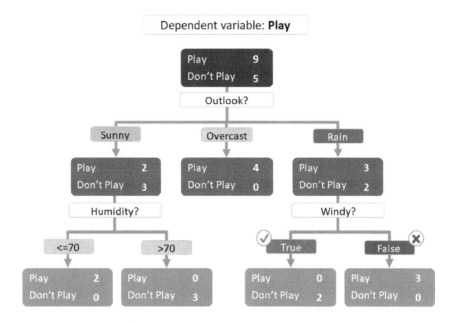

FIGURE 9.8.   Decision Tree as an Example of Graph-Based Learning

[sharief]. Each object or phenomenon becomes a node and each relationship an edge. Each relationship type is typically extracted to its own graph. All "preys upon" relationships will be analyzed separately.

Another luxury of GBL is being able to map graphs to sparse matrix operations [11]. Suppose a network has some labeled and some unlabeled nodes. For instance, if members of a population are known to be carriers of an allele. We can incorporate **label propagation** techniques to attempt to find new carriers. In this problem is modeled in terms of matrix decompositions so even extensive networks can be investigated.

GBL is only now starting to mature as the required computing power is becoming commonplace. The transparent coding and powerful mathematics make it another fascinating discipline of AI research.

INFORMATIONAL CAVE-INS

When people talk about variants of Artificial Intelligence, especially framed in the "Data Mining" brand, they bring up the notion of finding hidden patterns with the data. The belief is that your data has some correlation structure you haven't been able to tease out under standard methods. This is almost certainly true in any given data set and is probably tautological in dataset over a few thousand elements. Researchers scuttle quickly down into their data mines to extract these patterns, often unaware of the dangers.

Bonferroni Adjustments

Perhaps the most diabolical beast is neglecting to consider a Bonferroni adjustment. It is often ignored because it is very difficult to explain. The idea is that the more experiments you perform, the more likely you are to get a randomly "good" result.

The value is a common measure of a model's goodness of fit. In literature, a p-value of 0.05 or less suggests your model has captured actual information, and you're ready to publish! But let's not forget that your data has random noise within it, and that noise can accumulate to present as a correlation. The Bonferroni adjust suggests reducing your threshold p-value for the number of experiments run. A 0.95 confidence rate for one test would be increased to $1 - 0.5/2 = 0.975$ for two tests, $1 - 0.5/3 - 0.999$ for three. Each test would have satisfied this threshold.

In the world of big data, it is not uncommon to run thousands of tests. Thinking statistically, we could guess that at least 5% of all tests run are finding random, non-reproducible correlations, some of them with eye-poppingly positive results.

Data Collinearity

The topic of data collinearity is enormous, but researchers still manage to find ways to avoid noticing it. We talk about going into the data and uncovering hidden patterns, but so often we get tripped up by those same patterns.

This phenomenon is well studied in regression-based analyses like Linear, Logistic and Logit Regressions or Support Vector Machines, probably because the underlying linear algebra collapses when presented with collinear data. During the parameter fitting process, the data matrix is inverted—take 1 / Data—but this inverse only exists of no column of the data is a repeat or a multiple of another column.

This typically happens when one independent feature is implicitly influenced (or a function of) another independent feature. In Example [ex-kelp-forest], almost every variable is a function of the others, so the data is expected to be highly collinear.

Collinearity can mess up the models in multiple ways, the most obvious being that it just won't compute. Subtler is when the model oscillates between two solutions. If the features include something as obvious as **water column opacity** and 2 * **water column opacity**, the regression will simply pick one and lead you to falsely conclude 2 * **water column opacity** is the driving variable in kelp forest health.

Techniques such as Principle Component Analysis have been successful in removing co-linearity from the data set. This is standard practice for researchers using regression analysis. These structures are informative in and of themselves but are not generally seen as AI.

LET'S GO THERE

Technology and Artificial Intelligence are driven just as much by a hype cycle as any other business trend. In this chapter, I have attempted to illuminate the diaspora of techniques and the rich lineage within our field of Artificial Intelligence. I have presented bespoke definitions for otherwise opaque concepts and hope you find them useful.

It is not enough to subscribe to the fashions of AI, so we must strive to create new informational pathways. We can guide this exploration using an information-driven, Cybernetic framework. This is an exciting time! Regression was one of the first creatures to crawl ashore, balancing on the spindly legs of vector algebra. Information Theory grew out of its contact with the new landscape. Shortly after that the peculiar winner of the "Coolest Name" award, the Perceptron, was born, bringing a closer connection between biological and artificial systems. Time Series models grew eyes to look into the future, and Genetic Algorithms inspired a speciation event to rival the incredible life of the Burgess Shale. Now we enjoy the company of the Perceptron's grand-children, ANNs and Deep Learning, and we discover new relationships through Graph Based Learning. What will be next?

We are fortunate to be able to watch these systems chatter to themselves and each other. There is no common language, but messages are exchanged. How is this possible?

REFERENCES

1. Andrés, F., Galbraith, D. W., Talón, M., & Domingo, C. (2009). Analysis of PHOTO-PERIOD SENSITIVITY5 sheds light on the role of phytochromes in photoperiodic flowering in rice. *Plant Physiology, 109*, 681–690.
2. Liu, S., Ma, W., Moore, R., Ganesan, V., & Nelson, S. (2005). RxNorm: prescription for electronic drug information exchange. *IT Professional*. Retrieved from: https://www.computer.org/csdl/magazine/it/2005/05/f5017/13rRUxBa57X Vol 7
3. Webster, M. Artificial Intelligence. *Merriam-Webster*. Retrieved from: https://www.merriam-webster.com/dictionary/artificial%20intelligence.
4. Sutton, R., & Barto, A. (1998). *Reinforcement learning*. London, UK: MIT Press.
5. Gantz, J., & Reinse, D. (2012). The digital universe in 2020. *IDC iView*. Retrieved from: https://www.emc.com/leadership/digital-universe/2012iview/index.htm
6. Cox, D. (1958). The regression analysis of binary sequences (with discussion). *Journal of the Royal Statistical Society*. Retrieved from: https://www.nuffield.ox.ac.uk/users/cox/cox48.pdf Vol 20 No. 2
7. Rosenblatt, F. (1957). *The Perceptron—A perceiving and recognizing automaton*. Buffalo, NY: Cornell Aeronautical Laboratory.
8. Hinton, G., & Deng, L. (2009). *Deep learning for speech recognition and related applications*. Whistler, British Columbia: NIPS Workshops.
9. Holland, J. (1975). *Adaptation in natural and artificial systems*. London, UK: MIT Press.
10. Kolaczyk, E. (2009). *Statistical analysis of network data*. New York, NY: Springer.
11. Kepner, J., & Gilber, J. (2011). *Graph algorithms in the language of linear algebra*. Philadelphia, PA: SIAM.

ABOUT THE AUTHORS

Nathaniel Bischoff is currently a member of the data science team at Congoa Inc in Palo Alto, CA, a digital health platform company. He leverages deep learning techniques to analyze their unstructured data in the form of audio and video data to solve feature selection and classification problems. He previously was the Advanced Fellow in Artificial Intelligence in Medicine (AIMed) at Sharon Disney Lund Foundation's Medical Intelligence and Innovation Institute (MI3) at CHOC Children's in Orange, CA. Nathaniel has been fortunate enough to work with a number of passionate and talented multidisciplinary teams at Cognoa and CHOC including data scientists, engineers, physicians, and executives while collaborating with corporate and academic partners. Before joining MI3, Nathaniel was a part-time data analyst in Information Systems at CHOC Children's.

Nathaniel completed his Master of Sciences in Computational and Data Sciences with a focus in Bioinformatics at Chapman University's Schmid College of Science and Technology. He completed his Bachelor of Science in Biological Sciences with an emphasis in Computer Science and Informatics at the same institution. Nathaniel was a lead intern of MI3 Summer Internship during his undergraduate years. He is originally from Mountain View, CA. He shares the vision of many other pioneers in medical intelligence that data scientists and health care professionals must collaborate. Nathaniel is optimistic and confident that medical intelligence will amplify human intelligence to solve our biggest challenges in medicine.

Transforming Healthcare with Big Data and AI, pages 171–176.

Dr. Weixiang Chen currently serves as the Partner and California Chief Representative of Sinocapital Management, a global VC/PE company where she manages the high-tech investment in the US. Her investment interest primarily focuses on the applications of big data and AI in healthcare, manufacturing, and energy sector, where she sees tremendous demand for smart automation and digitalization. One area that she is especially interested in is digital health, since she firmly believes that technology is the ultimate solution to bring equal healthcare to everyone.

Dr. Chen holds a B.S. in Biological Science from Tsinghua University in China and a Ph.D. in Neuroscience from UCLA where she studied learning rules of artificial and physiological neural networks. She has worked as a data scientist in various companies, including a digital health startup. After that, she founded her own company to offer data-driven consulting services and apprenticeship-style data science training programs for graduate students.

Brian Dolan is well-known in the data community as a leading mathematician, data scientist, and cyberneticist with more than 20 years of hands-on experience. Prior to starting Verdant AI, Brian co-founded Deep 6 AI, Qurius Inc, and Discovix. Brian has consulted and led enterprise analytic projects from design to implementation for clients like EMC, SuperValu, Northern Trust, Zions National Bank, Havas Media, T-Mobile, the U.S. Intelligence Community, and Research In Motion. Formerly Chief Scientist at Greenplum (acquired by EMC), Brian also headed up data scientist teams at Yahoo! Inc. and served as Director of Research Analytics at FOX/MySpace.

Throughout his career, he has developed thousands of machine learning products, and his consulting clients include numerous state and local governments. He is also co-author of the seminal "MAD Skills: New Analysis Practices for Big Data," which has been cited more than 400 times in the big data/machine learning industry. In 2017 Brian spoke at TEDx Millsaps College on A Cybernetic View of AI in HealthCare Systems. Brian has a Master of Arts degree in Pure Mathematics from UCLA and a Master of Science degree in Bio-Mathematics from the David Geffen School of Medicine.

Alexandra Ehrlich is trained as a healthcare biostatistician and data scientist with over a decade of experience in epidemiology, clinical outcomes, clinical trials, and real-world evidence research. She holds a Master's in Public Health from the University of Florida specializing in Biostatistics and Epidemiology. She has led analytics efforts for a variety of programs at the Center for Disease Control (CDC), Southeastern Kaiser Permanente and Children's Healthcare of Atlanta.

Alexandra has an extensive background in informatics and data management technologies in healthcare and life sciences through roles at PerkinElmer Informatics and her current role with the Oracle Health Sciences Global Business Unit, where she performs a critical role as a thought leader for customers and the industry.

Dr. Atefeh (Anna) Farzindar is a research associate and Health Informatics advisor of the NSF's Integrated Media Systems Center (IMSC) and a faculty member of the Department of Computer Science, Viterbi School of Engineering at the University of Southern California (USC). She was the CEO and co-founder of NLP Technologies Inc., a company specializing in Natural Language Processing (NLP), established in Montreal, Canada and was the Adjunct Professor at University of Montreal.

Dr. Farzindar received her Ph.D. in Computer Science from the University of Montreal and her Master and Doctorate from Paris-Sorbonne University. She received Femmessor-Montréal awards, Succeeding with a balanced lifestyle, in the Innovative Technology and Information and Communications Technology category because of her involvement in the arts. Dr. Farzindar is a member of the Natural Sciences and Engineering Research Council of Canada (NSERC) Computer Science Liaison Committee and Member of the Canadian Advisory Committee of International Organization for Standardization (ISO).

Dr. Steve Garske is Senior Vice President and CIO at Children's Hospital Los Angeles. In this position, Steve leads a team of over 324 technical associates, physicians, and nurses and is responsible for managing all IT operational services for the system. Among their accomplishments, Steve and his current team have restructured IT management and suppliers in order to reduce operational costs while simultaneously increasing IT satisfaction rates.

Prior to his current work, Dr. Garske's experience includes serving as a CIO for Verity Health System, a CIO for Kootenai Health, a COO for Perot Systems Corporation at St. Joseph's Health System and an Account Executive for Computer Sciences Corporation. At Verity Health System, he helped create a 3-year IT strategic plan and was instrumental in launching initiatives to replace the entire network, consolidate data centers and servers, and provide a new WAN/LAN.

Dr. Garske is a results-driven healthcare technology leader with over ten years of CIO experience and over 20 years of technical experience. He is an expert in IT team building, major healthcare IT project implementations, EHR implementations, financial turnaround success, IT security, and new hospital building implementation. He holds a bachelor's degree in Applied Mathematics, Scientific Programming; a Master of Science Degree in Business IT, and a Ph.D. in Applied Management Decision Sciences, Information Systems Management. Steve is currently attending MIT (Massachusetts Institute of Technology) in Boston, Massachusetts (2017-2020) for his master's degree in Business Administration.

Cassandra Gibson is a UX designer with a background in biomedicine and medical humanities. Drawing on her specialized knowledge of healthcare and patient experience, Cassandra works with product teams and clients to bring life to problem-solving products. Cassandra has worked with a number of Sidebench clients, including Inland Empire Health Plan and the American Heart Association. She has also led workshops on topics such as user experience design, accessibility, and product strategy for TMCx, the healthcare startup accelerator in the Texas Medical Center and the WITH Foundation.

Mingbo Gong is an experienced technology consultant, currently working at Slalom Consulting, and previously at Deloitte Consulting and an LA-based healthcare consulting firm. Outside of consulting, he is an angel investor at the Pasadena Angels Group and serves as an advisory board member at two digital healthcare startups. Mingbo is also the founder of SixThirty Group, a 501(c)(3) nonprofit incubator that focuses on the intersection of open data, smart cities, and digital healthcare. Through founding SixThirty Group, he was recognized by the California State Assembly for "exemplary leadership" in driving digital innovations.

Mingbo received an M.S. degree in Business Analytics from the University of Southern California and B.S. degrees in Accounting Information Systems and Business Administration from the same institution.

Hugh Gordon is a practicing physician and veteran software engineer with expertise in security and infrastructure engineering. He started his career at Google, eventually serving as the tech lead on the team that rebuilt Google's single sign-on infrastructure. Hugh left Google in order to pursue a career in medicine, and during his medical school training, he co-founded Akido Labs, Inc., a healthcare data management company and served as Chief Technology Officer. Hugh has since returned to clinical medicine and now works as a physician at LAC+USC medical center. He also serves as a founder of and advisor to USC's Digital Health Lab, which helps eliminate roadblocks to technical innovation in the healthcare system. Hugh received his B.S. in computer engineering from Columbia University and his MD from USC's Keck School of Medicine.

Kenneth Hayashida Jr. is a board-certified and licensed pediatrician and is adjunct faculty at the Keck School of Medicine of USC mentoring student teams in the Health, Technology, & Engineering Program. As a community-based pediatrician, Ken was on medical staff at multiple community hospitals, provided care to thousands of newborns, infants, and children, and maintained contracting with most major health insurers in California and Hawaii. Ken is also a founding member of the I3 Consortium at USC, where he is contributing definition and thought to the medical use cases of IoT infrastructure and data.

With a degree in Biological Sciences with Honors from the University of Southern California, Ken was President of the USC Alpha Alpha chapter of the Phi Sigma National Biological Sciences Honor Society. He was chosen by NASA for the 1988 Space Life Sciences Training Program at Kennedy Space Center where he received training from NASA astronauts, physicians, and life scientists.

Ken has a Doctor of Medicine from the Keck School of Medicine of USC and completed internship and residency at the Children's Hospital of Orange County.

While served as the residency program representative to the American Academy of Pediatrics Section on Residents, Ken was selected for national executive committee service for the Section on Computing and Other Technologies, was present in the early definition of digital communication standards for pediatrics, contributed definition to electronic medical records, and was the editor of the section newsletter for a year.

Dr. Diana Inkpen is a Professor at the University of Ottawa, in the School of Electrical Engineering and Computer Science. She obtained her Ph.D. from the University of Toronto, Department of Computer Science. She has an M.Sc. and B.Eng. degree in Computer Science and Engineering from the Technical University of Cluj-Napoca, Romania. Her research is in the applications of Natural Language Processing and Text Mining. She organized seven international workshops and was a program co-chair for the 25th Canadian Conference on Artificial Intelligence conference. She is also the editor-in-chief of the Computational Intelligence journal and an associate editor for the Natural Language Engineering journal.

Dr. Inkpen was an invited speaker for the Applied Natural Language Processing track at the 29th Florida Artificial Intelligence Research Society Conference, for the 28th Canadian Conference on Artificial Intelligence, and International Symposium on Information Management and Big Data. She published a book on Natural Language Processing for Social Media (Morgan and Claypool Publishers, Synthesis Lectures on Human Language Technologies, the second edition appeared in 2017), nine book chapters, more than 30 journal articles, and more than 100 conference papers. She received many research grants, from which the majority include intensive industrial collaborations.

Dr. Alex Liu is a chief data scientist at IBM Analytics Services. Before joined IBM in 2013, he served as a chief data scientist or lead data scientist for a few companies including Ingram Micro, Yapstone, and iSKY. Dr. Liu taught advanced data analytics at the University of Southern California and the University of California, Irvine as an adjunct professor, while he also consulted for organizations like the United Nations. He has a Ph.D. of Quantitative Sociology and an M.S. of Statistical Computing from Stanford University.

Dr. Liu's special data science approach centers on bringing up positive social impacts with technologies, for which he received many awards, including the Outstanding Service Award from the Graduate Student Association in USA, the Nonprofit Campaign Award from the Media Alliance, the outstanding service award from USAID, the AIU teaching innovation award, the IBM Solution award, the IBM Hero award, and the Fulbright Fellowship.

Benjamin Nguyen. Prior to joining Sidebench, Ben Nguyen worked at the USC Center for Body Computing, a digital health research division. His projects involved everything from virtual human avatars to mobile chronic disease management. Ben's experience combines the worlds of medicine, technology, and business - starting with medical training at the USC Keck School of Medicine and work at both the USC Viterbi School of Engineering and the USC Marshall School of Business. At Sidebench, Ben leads healthcare product strategy to deliver value to clients such as Inland Empire Health, Children's Hospital Los Angeles, and Los Angeles County DCFS.

Jerry Power is the Executive Director of The Institute for Communication Technology Management (CTM) at the University of Southern California's Marshall School of Business. CTM is actively engaged in identifying, understanding, and leveraging emerging trends driven by the rapid evolution of digital communications technologies and services. Through CTMs research and educational programs, the Institute explores the new opportunities and challenges in the age of digital transformations. CTM embraces our increasingly dynamic market and harnesses the thought leadership of the University and the CTM community to find new ways to thrive in this evolving business climate.

Jerry is also a founding member of the I3 Consortium. I3 is working to create an open source Internet-of-Things data governance tool that allows communities of independent IOT device owners to work together as active members of the expanding data ecosystem. The consortium recognizes the importance and the personalized nature of privacy, trust, and incentives as key enablers of a sustainable, managed, and networked IOT infrastructure that supports collaborative IOT environments where data must transcend organization boundaries.

Jerry is also the co-author of a book to be coming out August 2019 entitled "The Real Time Revolution: Transforming your organization to value customer Time."

Kevin Yamazaki is the Founder & CEO of Sidebench, an award-winning digital product and venture studio based in Los Angeles. He has extensive experience in management and technology consulting having worked as a technology advisor to the Mayor of Honolulu and as a senior technology consultant at Accenture. While at Accenture, Kevin built his knowledge of user experience & product design through working with Disney Studio's R&D and Strategy & Innovation Groups. Kevin is an angel investor, a start-up advisor and volunteers on the board and committees for several non-profits, including MSMF (suicide prevention) and the Children's Hospital of Los Angeles. Kevin was recognized on the Forbes 30 Under 30 list for his work in building Sidebench, which was recently recognized on the Inc. 500 as one of the fastest-growing companies in America.